Renal Radiology and Imaging

O. P. FitzGerald-Finch, MB, BS, FRCR

Consultant Radiologist, Glasgow Royal Infirmary, Glasgow

Published,
in association with
UPDATE PUBLICATIONS LTD., by

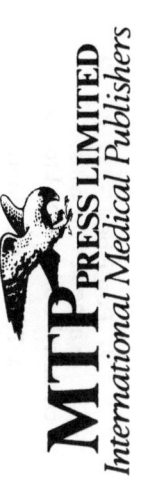

MTP **PRESS LIMITED**
International Medical Publishers

Published,
in association with
Update Publications Ltd., by

MTP Press Limited
Falcon House
Lancaster, England

Copyright © 1981 MTP Press Limited

First published 1981

ISBN-13: 978-94-009-8074-7   e-ISBN-13: 978-94-009-8072-3
DOI: 10.1007/978-94-009-8072-3

Softcover reprint of the hardcover 1st edition 1981

Contents

Acknowledgements

Many colleagues have provided radiographs for this book. I am deeply indebted to the following: Dr F. G. Adams (Figures 5.2, 5.3, 10.4), Dr D. Briggs (Figure 10.7), Dr P. Crumlish (Figure 1.2), Dr J. K. Davidson (Figures 6.3, 9.5, 10.12), Dr S. Davidson (Figures 3.6, 3.10, 4.11, 4.12, 7.5, 9.1), Dr H. Gray (Figures 1.11, 7.14, 8.4), Dr W. James (Figures 1.3, 1.9, 3.5, 4.3, 4.6, 4.10, 4.14, 5.1, 6.5, 6.6, 7.4, 7.9, 8.3, 9.2, 9.4), Dr L. Kreel (Figure 8.1), Dr G. McCreath (Figure 3.9), Dr P. Morley (Figures 4.2, 10.8, 10.9), Dr E. Sweet (Figures 3.1, 3.3, 4.13).

Introduction

Considerable changes have taken place in the investigation of renal disease since the time when the two basic radiographic examinations were the intravenous pyelogram (IVP) and retrograde studies. Better understanding of the normal and pathophysiology, improved contrast reagents and modern technology have now greatly increased the diagnostic scope and accuracy of urinary tract investigation.

An investigation sequence can now be planned in order to make the diagnosis in the minimum time while sparing the patient possibly unpleasant and potentially hazardous examinations. A good example of this is in the investigation of a renal 'mass' found on intravenous urography (IVU).

Clinical fashions change and this is reflected in the demands made on ancillary departments, as has happened in the investigation of renovascular hypertension.

The subject of this book is the kidney and this will form the bulk of the subject matter but, of course, renal tract pathology affects and is affected by diseases in other systems and elsewhere in the renal tract, and, where relevant, examples will be discussed.

1. Methods of Investigation

In this chapter the principal methods of investigation of the kidney will be discussed. The indications, contraindications and limitations of the various procedures will be described and, where relevant, the normal anatomy will be outlined. Detailed descriptions of the techniques of individual examinations will not be described as these can be found in any standard text book. However, practical points of clinical significance will be illustrated.

Intravenous Urography (IVU)

The IVU remains the standard primary examination in the investigation of renal disease with only two major contraindications—pregnancy and known allergy to contrast agents. Incipient cardiac failure and myeloma are relative contraindications. It is now considered safe to carry out an IVU in patients with myeloma as long as preliminary dehydration is avoided. Any doctor who injects contrast agents must question the patient concerning previous reactions to contrast agents and other

allergies. He should also familiarize himself with the treatment of allergic reactions (Sutton and Grainger 1975) and ensure that adequate resuscitation equipment and drugs are available.

Patients are normally prepared with a course of aperients and 12 hours dehydration. Dehydration is contraindicated in renal failure and, as noted above, should not be used in patients with myeloma.

Prior to the injection of a contrast agent, a plain film must be taken, with oblique views if necessary, to demonstrate calcified opacities which may be subsequently obscured (Figure 1.1). The contrast agents are tri-iodinated compounds and a dose equivalent to 16 g of iodine is injected. The actual contrast agent used is relatively unimportant although it has been shown that for an equivalent dose a slightly greater contrast density in the pelvicalyceal system will be achieved with sodium rather than meglumine.

The contrast agents are excreted mainly by glomerular filtration and to a small extent by tubular excretion. Less than one per cent is normally excreted through the alternative pathways, which are mainly the liver and small intestine (Figure 1.2).

A typical examination consists of a five-minute film without compression to show the pelvicalyceal system, a ten-minute film with compression (Figure 1.3a and b), and films of the full and empty bladder to show any residual volume.

3

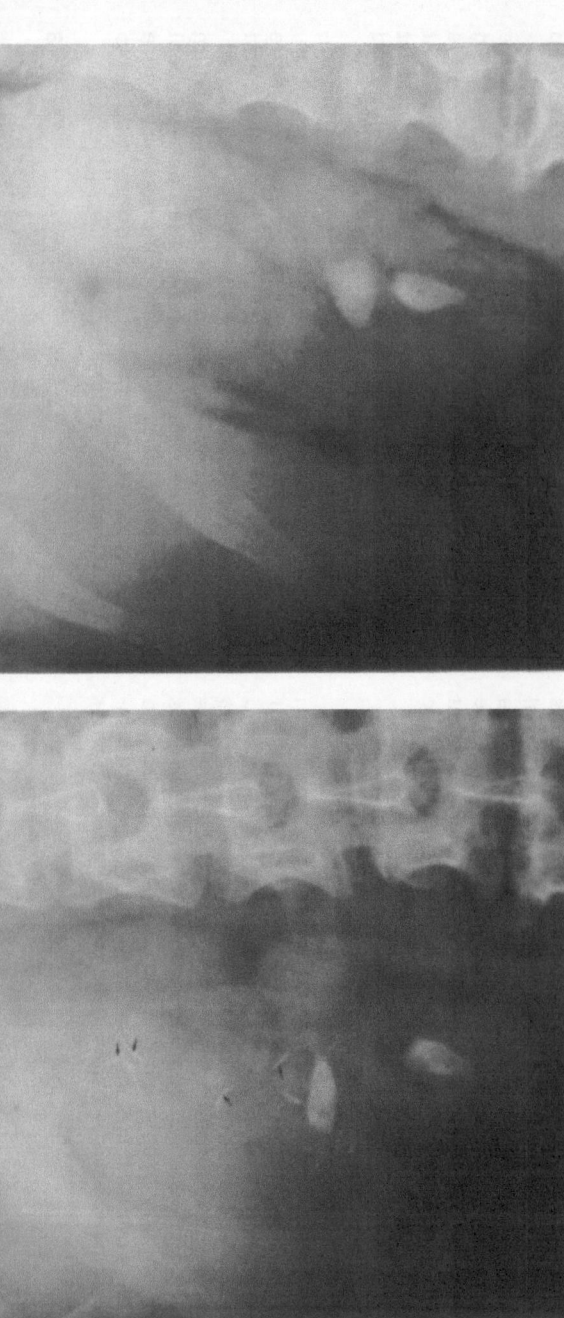

Figure 1.1. **(a)** *On the straight film there are multiple linear densities projected over the right kidney (arrowed) in addition to the two renal calculi.* **(b)** *The oblique film confirms that these are gall stones.*

In the investigation of hypertension early sequence films are taken at one and two minutes. If compression is contraindicated or not tolerated, a compromise is to tilt the patient's head down.

Inspiration/expiration films may be required to assess the relationship of calcified opacities to the pelvicalyceal systems or ureters and in certain circumstances to demonstrate immobility of a kidney, e.g.

patient is turned prone and left for three or four minutes before the radiograph is taken in order to allow the contrast to diffuse to the level of the obstruction. Delayed films of up to 24 hours may also be necessary.

Zonography (short tube swing tomography) is very valuable when overlying bowel loops are obscuring the kidneys (Figure 1.4a and b).

Water Load

Giving a water load after an IVU examination will exaggerate the differential excretion rate of contrast in renovascular hypertension. A water load can also be used to precipitate pelviureteric obstruction and is usually followed by an intravenous injection of frusemide or a similar diuretic (Figure 1.5).

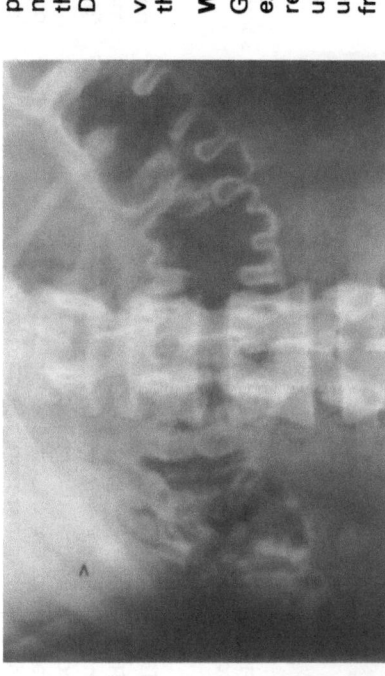

Figure 1.2 *Excretion of contrast via the liver. Note the contrast filled gall bladder (arrowhead) and the contrast lining the bowel wall.*

with a renal abscess. Two exposures are made on the same film and if there is localized inflammatory disease, the affected kidney will be 'splinted' and will not move while the unaffected one will be blurred by movement.

In the investigation of obstruction, prone films can be very useful to demonstrate the level of obstruction. The

The Nephrogram

The nephrogram results from contrast in the proximal collecting tubules and is independent of hydration. The density of the nephrogram depends on the injected dose and will also be maximal at the end of a bolus injection of contrast. A bolus injection will give better results in nephrotomography than an infusion (which will not achieve such high plasma and therefore glomerular filtrate concentrations).

Kelsey et al. (1972) have described three main types of abnormal nephrogram which will be described later.

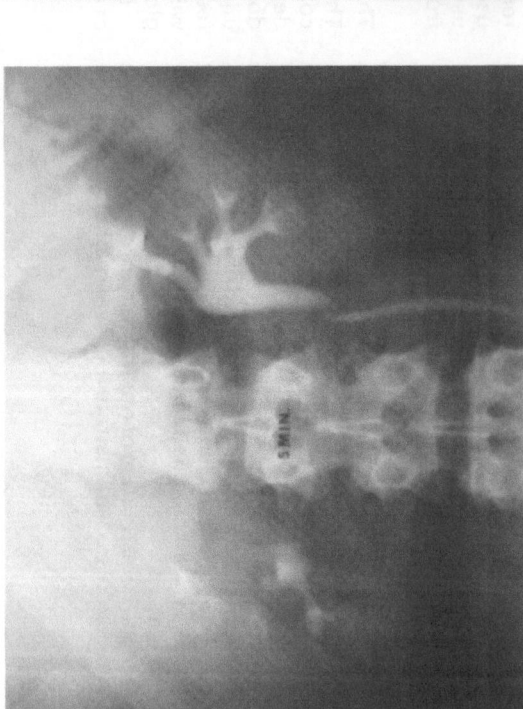

Figure 1.3. *IVU with compression.* (a) *The five-minute film shows an apparent filling defect in the right kidney, but after compression at 10 minutes* (b), *this is excluded.*

The Pyelogram

The pyelogram depends on the density of the collecting systems, which is proportional to the amount of contrast within the collecting units. This, among other factors, depends on the activity of antidiuretic hormone and is therefore affected by dehydration, unlike a nephrogram. The pyelographic density is affected by many other factors and is thus a poor guide to renal function.

In paediatric practice, a useful manoeuvre to clear overlying bowel from the kidneys, particularly the left, is to give a carbonated drink following the contrast

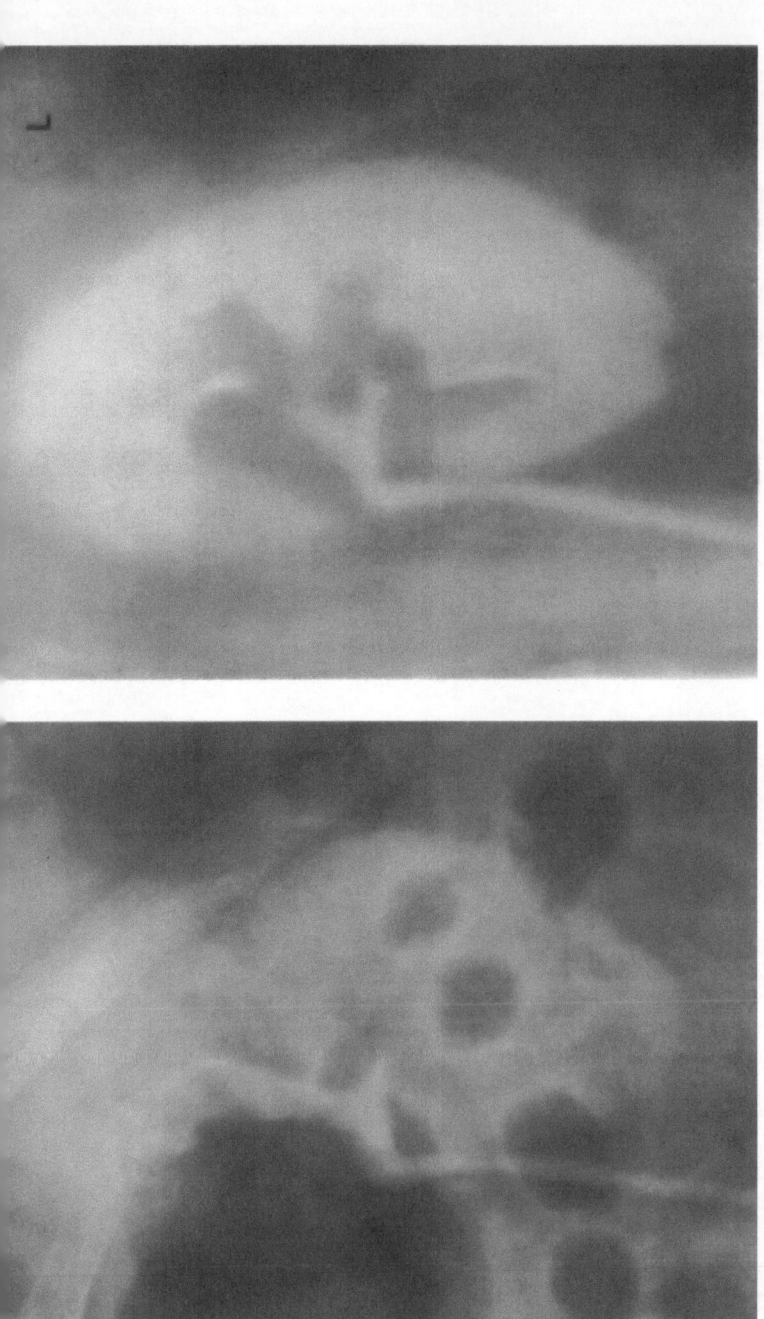

Figure 1.4 *Effects of tomography.* **(a)** *View of the kidney obscured by abdominal gases.* **(b)** *Kidney revealed by zonography.*

injection so that the stomach will be distended by gas and act as a window through which the left kidney can be seen.

Renal Anatomy

The normal adult kidney has a long diameter between 11 and 14cm, or a length equivalent to L2 plus the disc L2–3 × 3 to 3.5.

On a pyelogram a line joining the tips of the renal papillae bears a constant relationship to the margin of the kidney, the distance between the two representing the renal substance.

Retrograde Pyelogram

The indications are:

1. The localization of obstructing lesions and their cause, if this has not been demonstrated by other means.

2. The demonstration of ureteric lesions.

3. The clarification of renal lesions where IVU has been unsatisfactory.

4. Rarely, in renal failure to exclude obstruction when high dose studies have been unsuccessful.

Retrograde examinations should not be carried out blindly, but should be monitored with fluoroscopy so that the taking of films can be timed and overfilling avoided. The patient can be appropriately rotated

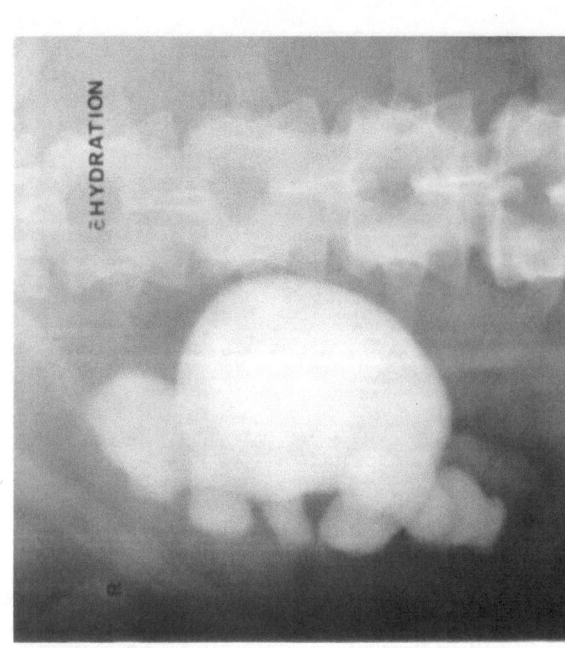

Figure 1.5. Pelviureteric obstruction in a female patient with intermittent right loin pain in whom the initial IVU was reported as normal. Infusion IVU with hydration has precipitated the pelviureteric hold-up.

when the location of opacities is uncertain, and use of a videotape is of value when peristaltic function is clinically important.

The hazards of the examination include instrumental perforation, infection, ureteric obstruction due to oedema and contrast extravasation (Figure 1.6).

Pyelotubular Extravasation

Pyelotubular extravasation is a common, normal finding which is exaggerated by compression and retrograde injection, and appears as fine linear opacities radiating from the minor calyces. The major differential diagnoses are medullary sponge kidney and an early tuberculous lesion.

The varying degrees of true extravasation have been named according to the anatomical location of the contrast: pyelosinus, peripelvic, pyelolymphatic, pyelovenous and pyelointerstitial extravasation.

Many other causes of extravasation have been described, the commonest being calculus obstruction of the ureter. The list also includes other causes of ureteric obstruction, e.g. neoplasm and surgical ligation, polycystic kidney and tumour of the renal pelvis.

Antegrade Pyelogram

Antegrade pyelography examination is occasionally of value when IVU has not established the site of an obstructing lesion, and a retrograde is either undesir-

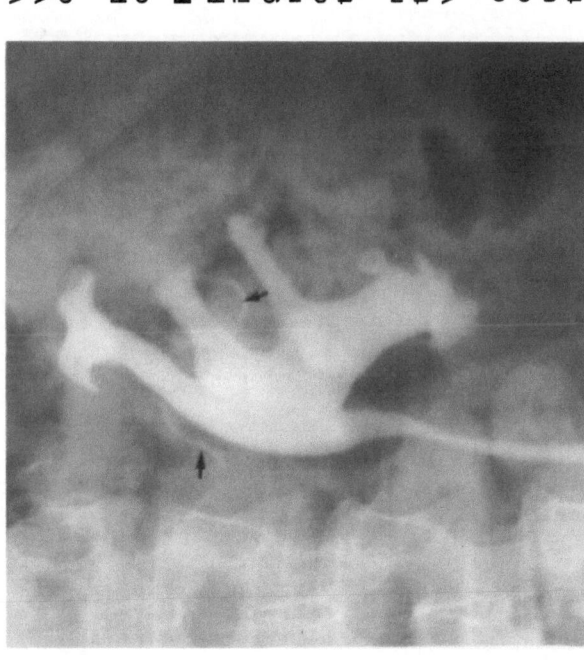

Figure 1.6. Pyelolymphatic extravasation during retrograde study in a patient with a large hypernephroma. Curvilinear tracks of contrast are spreading out from the upper calyces (arrowed).

9

able or impossible, for example when an ileal conduit has been established.

The examination can be carried out either under screen control following high dose IVU or under ultrasound or computerized tomography (CT) control. After the introduction of contrast the patient is, if necessary, put in the erect position to establish the level of obstruction and the cannula can remain in situ as a draining nephrostomy (Figure 1.7).

Cyst Puncture

Renal cyst puncture now forms an integral part of the investigation of a renal 'mass' found on IVU. Like antegrade pyelography, it can be carried out immediately following the intravenous urogram (Figure 1.8) or under ultrasound or CT control. The part played by cyst puncture is dealt with more fully in chapter 4.

Vascular Studies

Angiography

A main stream aortogram should always be carried out prior to selective renal studies to exclude contralateral pathology and to establish the anatomy. Multiple renal arteries are a common normal variant (Figure 1.9), and bizarre and misleading appearances can result if a selective study is carried out without a prior main stream angiogram.

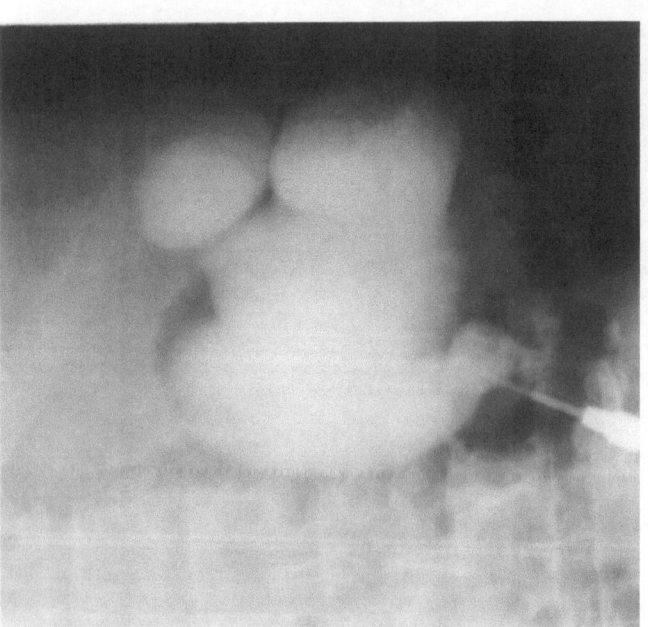

Figure 1.7. Antegrade pyelogram. Large non-functioning left kidney thought to be due to hydronephrosis resulting from a calculus. An antegrade pyelogram confirmed this, and the cannula was left in as a draining nephrostomy.

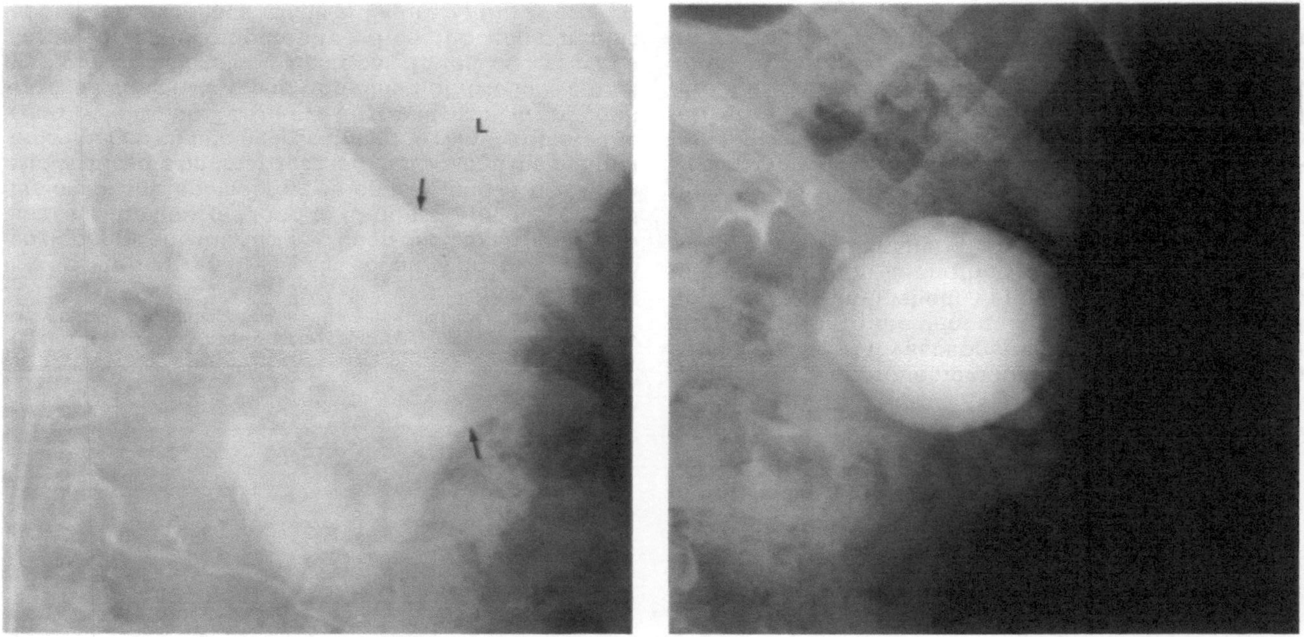

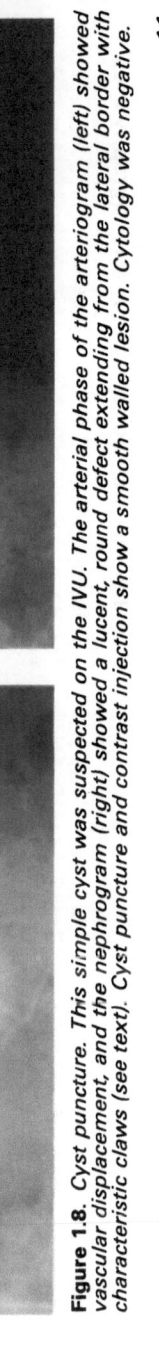

Figure 1.8. Cyst puncture. This simple cyst was suspected on the IVU. The arterial phase of the arteriogram (left) showed vascular displacement, and the nephrogram (right) showed a lucent, round defect extending from the lateral border with characteristic claws (see text). Cyst puncture and contrast injection show a smooth walled lesion. Cytology was negative.

The principal indications for arteriography are:

1. Investigation of renal masses.
2. Renovascular hypertension.
3. Trauma.
4. Transplant malfunction.
5. A non-functioning kidney.
6. Small vessel disease.
7. Unexplained haematuria.

Venography

Considerable improvement in intrarenal venous filling can be achieved if vasoconstrictors are injected intra-arterially prior to the venous injection when the renal flow will be diminished. Venous occlusion using an inflatable balloon is another method of reducing the rapid venous drainage.

Micturating Cystogram

Recent work (Hodson et al. 1975) has shown a connection between the presence of vesicoureteric reflux with intrarenal reflux and the subsequent formation of atrophic pyelonephritis and renal scarring. Therefore, when micturating cystography is carried out, it is important to determine whether intrarenal reflux is present or not (see Figure 3.3).

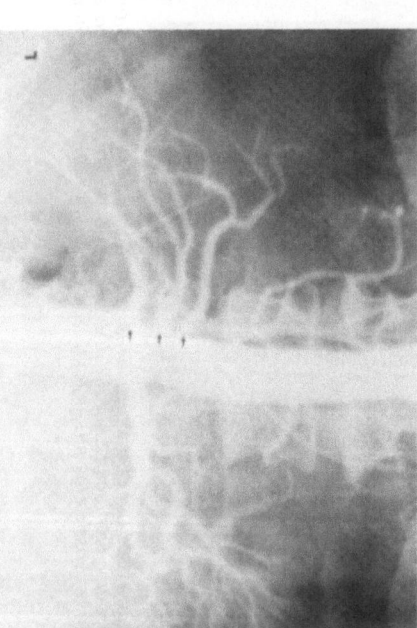

Figure 1.9. *Three renal arteries supplying the left kidney, which is hydronephrotic.*

The normal renal vessels constrict in response to epinephrine and this fact has been used to advantage to increase the flow of blood to tumours. The dosage and timing of the epinephrine is critical, and it has been shown that the optimal dose is 2 to 5 µg, and the optimal time interval should be less than one minute before the contrast injection. Too high a dose will result in proximal vascular constriction and non-filling of distal intrarenal vessels. Occasionally it has been found necessary to carry out angiotomography when the angiographic appearances are inconclusive (Figure 1.10).

Isotopes

Isotope studies which can detect overall and divided renal function provide an essential complement to conventional contrast studies which are an unreliable method of assessing renal function.

A normal density can be seen on IVU with a renal function reduced to 20 per cent of normal. The pyelographic density can be reduced if excess fluid intake precedes the examination, and the density will increase if the kidney is ischaemic or obstructed. Twenty per cent of patients with renovascular hypertension will have a normal pyelogram. Conversely, renal artery stenosis can be shown on angiography in patients who are hypertensive but have no other evidence that this is due to renovascular causes. On the other hand, renography provides a reliable screening procedure for renovascular hypertension.

The other principal uses of isotope studies are in paediatrics where more invasive and potentially hazardous procedures, such as cystoscopy, can be avoided; in the diagnosis, assessment and follow-up of obstruction; in trauma; in the assessment of transplant function; and in patients with a known allergy to contrast media.

The three main imaging techniques referable to the renal tract are:

1. Static renal imaging.

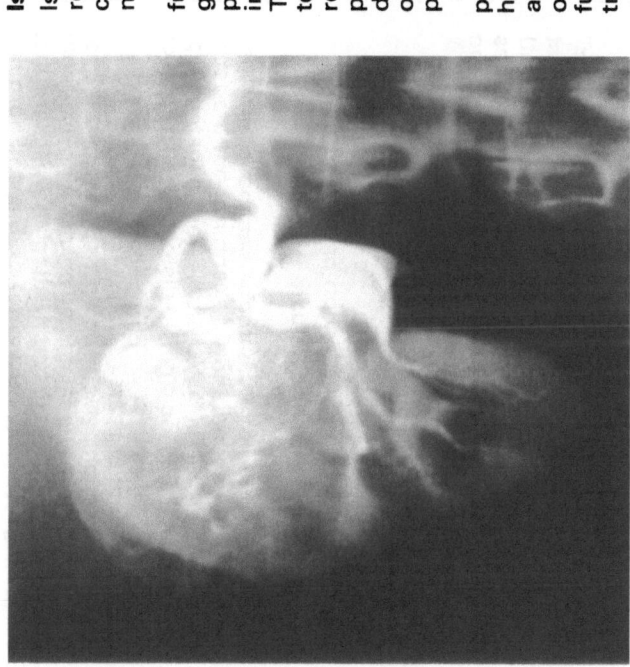

Figure 1.10. *Angionephrotomography in a case of hypernephroma. The tomographic cut was taken during a selective angiogram.*

13

2. Renography.

3. Reflux studies.

Static Renal Imaging

The commonest radiopharmaceutical used is $^{99}Tc^m$ DMSA (dimercaptosuccinic acid), which is almost completely taken up by the parenchyma (97 per cent) after intravenous injection. Gamma camera pictures are taken at four hours postinjection (Figure 1.11). The technique has four main uses:

1. Anatomical studies of parenchymal lesions.

2. Divided function studies.

3. Intrarenal division of function prior to surgery.

4. In iodine-sensitive individuals.

The demonstration of anatomy has been replaced largely by ultrasound and CT scanning, but the technique remains useful if IVU studies are negative (e.g. with a lesion that is too small to distort either calyces or the renal margin) or equivocal, and to confirm pseudotumours or scars.

Divided function, which should be 50 per cent + 2 per cent in each kidney, is calculated by counting over both kidneys separately and subtracting the background. The findings are only relevant if drainage is normal.

Renography

The commonly used radiopharmaceuticals, which are rapidly excreted by glomerular filtration, are $^{99}Tc^m$ DTPA (diethylene tetramine penta-acetic acid) and ^{131}I hippuran.

The information is presented in two ways:

1. A time/activity curve of each kidney, which is a 'renogram' from which background activity has been subtracted (Figure 1.12).

2. Gamma camera pictures.

If a probe is sited over the heart, a figure for the renal input, following intravenous injection, can be obtained.

Diuresis Renography

Diuresis renography is normally performed following a standard renogram. Prior to the second injection of the radio-pharmaceutical, the patient is given a large fluid load, followed by an intravenous diuretic, such as frusemide. The renogram is then repeated.

On the standard renogram, both a hypotonic renal pelvis and a true obstruction will give an 'obstructive pattern', i.e. a continuously rising phase II without a peak or phase III. Following diuresis, however, the hypotonic pelvis will show a third phase descent on the renogram, while the true obstruction will be unaltered.

Retention Function Studies

If a computer with 'region of interest' facility is available, it is possible to calculate the rate of passage through, or the abnormal retention of the isotope in, the whole kidney and the parenchyma. Renal function

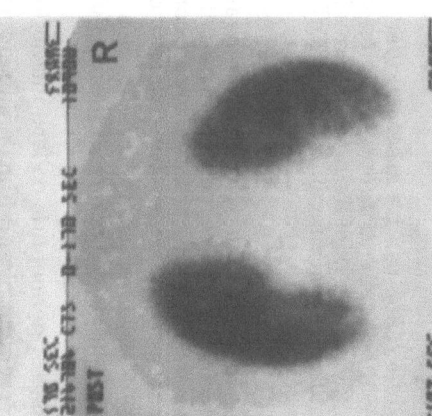

Figure 1.12. The normal renogram is divided into three phases. Phase 1 takes place within 30 seconds of the injection and represents the arrival of the radiopharmaceutical in the kidney, renal vessels and perirenal tissues. Phase 2 represents the accumulation of the radiopharmaceutical in the kidney. Phase 3 follows the peak and represents drainage.

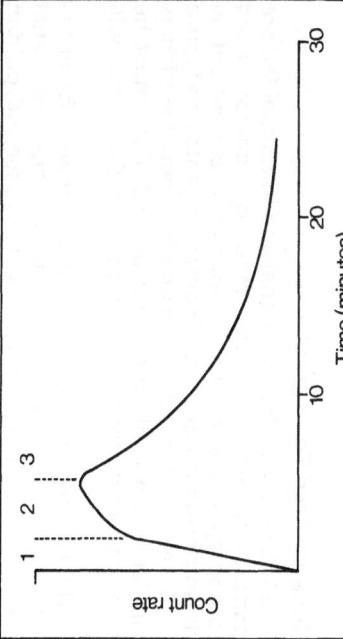

Figure 1.11. Normal parenchymal study of both kidneys using ⁹⁹Tcᵐ DMSA.

15

(RF) studies are used in, for example, obstruction and suspected renovascular disease.

Reflux Studies

Vesicoureteric reflux can be assessed (particularly in children) without catheterization by doing a gamma camera study during micturition following the excretion of a radiopharmaceutical, such as $^{99}Tc^m$ DTPA.

Ultrasound

Ultrasound is a completely safe, non-invasive procedure, which now forms an essential part of the diagnostic work up of renal masses used in conjunction with diagnostic cyst puncture. The other principal uses of ultrasound are:

1. Identifying fluid collections in association with a renal transplant.

2. Diagnosis of perinephric collections of fluid.

3. The assessment of non-functioning kidneys.

4. The demonstration of hydronephrosis.

5. Showing renal position and size.

6. The diagnosis of polycystic disease.

7. Monitoring renal size in renal failure.

8. Examination of kidneys in pregnancy and in patients with contrast sensitivity.

The kidneys are normally scanned with the patient prone, although the right kidney is often well seen through the liver shadow in the supine position and, if the spleen is enlarged, the left kidney can similarly be shown. Figure 1.13 shows the normal ultrasonic renal anatomy.

Computerized Tomography

The kidneys, with their perirenal and intrarenal fat, are particularly well demonstrated by computerized tomography, and enhancement can be carried out by the intravenous injection of contrast agents (see Figure 4.15 a and b). If a bolus injection is given, the effect is similar to the nephrogram on an IVU. Care must be taken to avoid movement, or 'streaking' artefacts will result.

The CT measurement of density allows differentiation of, for instance, haematoma, abscess, renal tumour or hydronephrosis. As with ultrasound, guided biopsy and cyst puncture can be carried out. Figure 1.14 shows the normal CT anatomy of the kidneys.

The principal uses of the technique are:

1. Investigation of the non-functioning kidney.

2. Investigation of renal and perirenal masses (Figure 1.15).

3. Remote pathology.

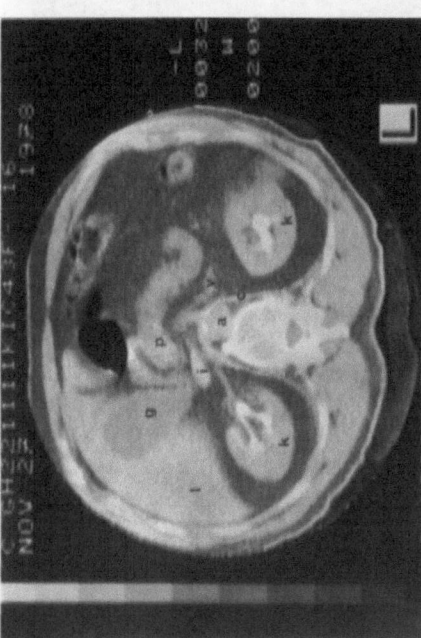

Figure 1.14. *CT scan. Normal anatomy through kidneys. l, liver; g, gall bladder; p, pancreas; i, inferior vena cava; a, aorta giving off the right renal artery and, anteriorly, the superior mesenteric artery; v, left renal vein; c, crura of diaphragm; k, kidney. The dark tissue is fat.*

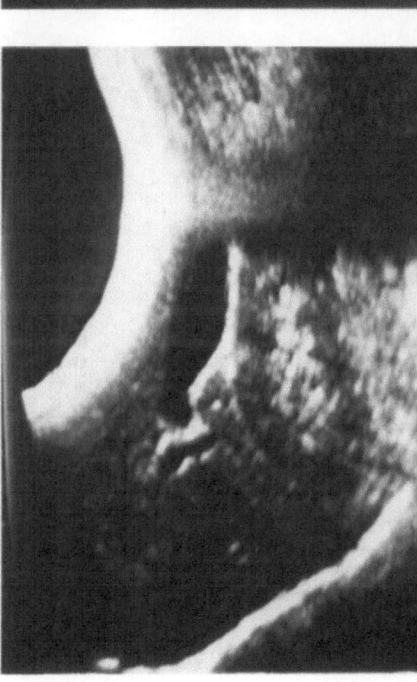

Figure 1.13. *Ultrasound. Normal longitudinal scan of right kidney.*

Two dimensional reconstruction may help in deciding whether a mass arises from the kidney.

Renal Radiography in Pregnancy

Radiography is contraindicated in pregnancy, but, if it is performed, then it can be shown that there is bilateral hydroureter and hydronephrosis (Figure 1.16). This returns to normal in approximately 14 weeks, although with multiple pregnancies the return may be less than

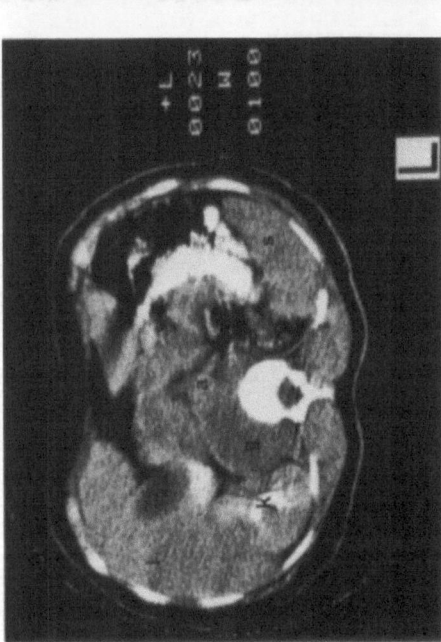

Figure 1.15. *CT scan. Displacement of the right kidney by a glandular mass in a female patient, aged 26 years, with lymphoma. Scan shows large mass of glands (g) displacing right kidney (k); s, spleen; a, aorta; l, liver.*

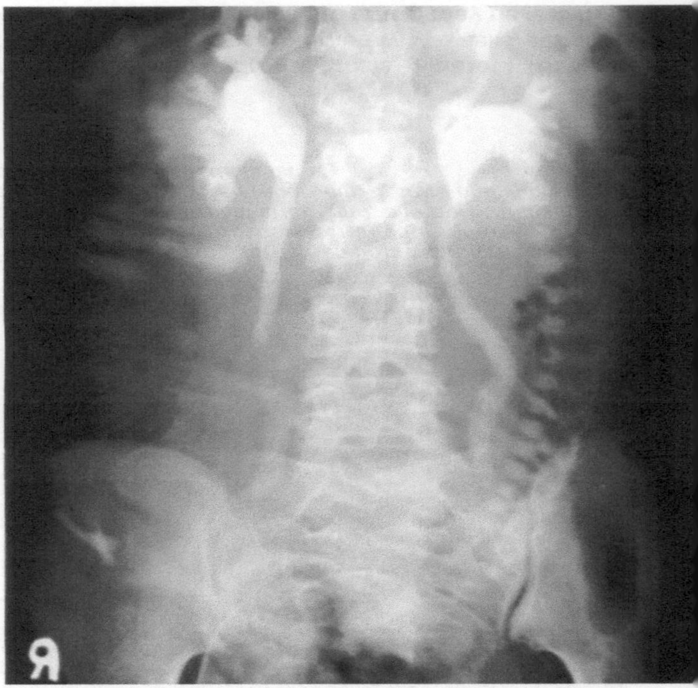

Figure 1.16. *Hydroureter and hydronephrosis in pregnancy.*

complete. The changes are more marked on the right and any postpartum radiographic studies should be delayed, if possible, for approximately 14 weeks, so that true disease can be assessed.

2. Congenital Variations

Renal Dysplasia

The kidneys in renal dysplasia are usually four to five centimetres in length and have dilated calyces. The principal differential diagnosis is from chronic pyelonephritis, which will show the characteristic scarring. The other form of renal dysplasia is the unilateral multicystic kidney (see Chapter 5, page 45). The diagnostic features are:

1. The kidney is non-functioning.

2. There is an absent or rudimentary renal artery.

3. There is an absent or atretic ureter.

4. CT and ultrasound will show multiple cystic spaces.

Agenesis

Renal venography has been shown to be a useful way of distinguishing a small contracted kidney from agenesis. In agenesis there will be only a renal vein and non-renal, for example, gonadal, tributaries whereas in a small contracted kidney a diminished renal vein with the corresponding renal lobar veins will be demonstrated.

A contrast enhanced CT study will also help the physician to make the diagnosis.

Hypoplasia

The main differential diagnosis is from postobstructive atrophy, where there will be dilated calyces. A hypoplastic kidney has a reduced number of calyces.

Ectopia

The commonest site for an ectopic kidney is within the pelvis, and, if contrast studies are inconclusive, enhanced CT is a useful method of demonstrating a pelvic kidney.

Ectopic kidneys can also occur in the thorax, where they are normally in the lower thorax on the left side and are usually detected as an incidental finding. They function normally.

Crossed-Ectopia

The ectopic kidney is usually malrotated and fused with the opposite kidney (Figure 2.1). Rotation can, of course, occur in normally sited kidneys.

Fusion—Horseshoe Kidney

Horseshoe kidney is the commonest form of renal fusion and, as with other congenital abnormalities,

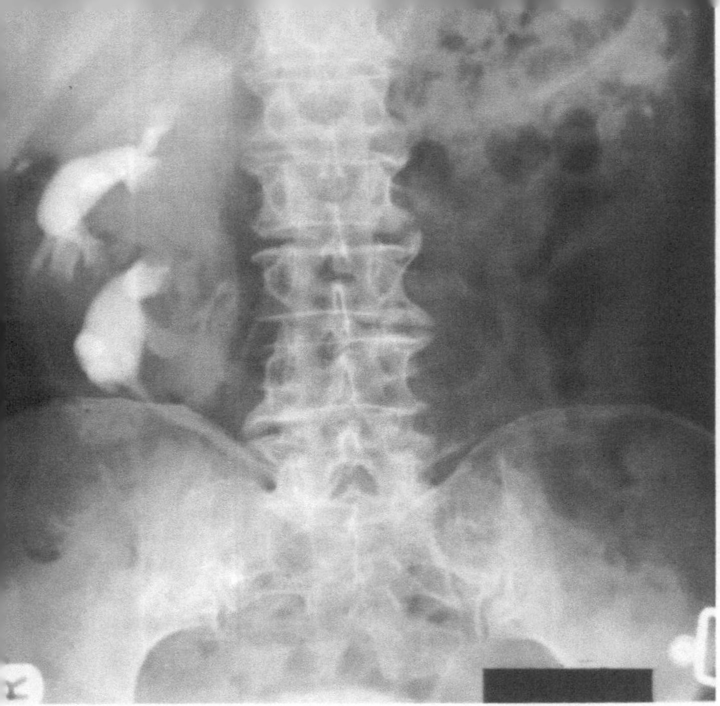

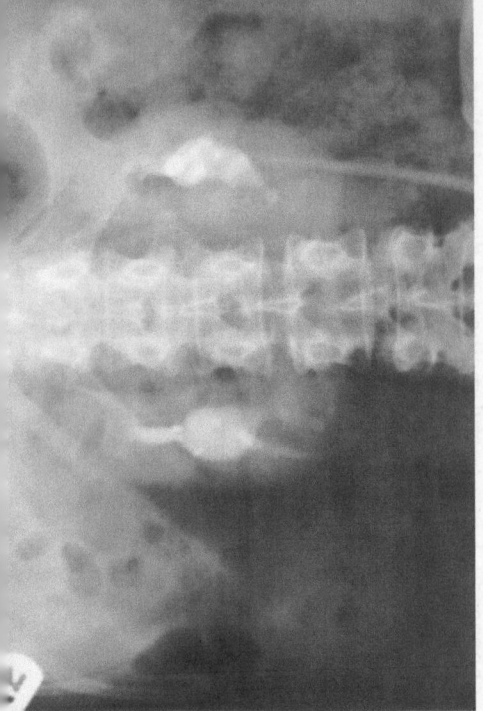

Figure 2.2. Horseshoe kidney. Note the vertical alignment of the two (fused) kidneys. Both kidneys are rotated and the ureters arise anteriorly.

there is a higher incidence of complications such as calculus formation, pyelonephritis and hydronephrosis. Hydronephrosis has been shown to occur in up to a third of patients affected; it is caused by pelviureteric obstruction and it is associated with rotation. Rotation can vary from the normal laterally pointing calyces to a posterolateral location, and, in the extreme

Figure 2.1. Right-sided unilateral fused kidney.

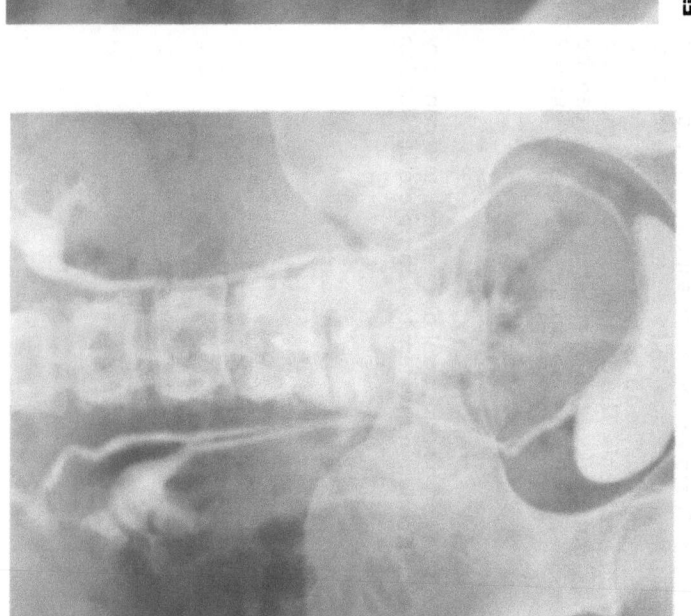

Figure 2.3. Duplex right collecting system.

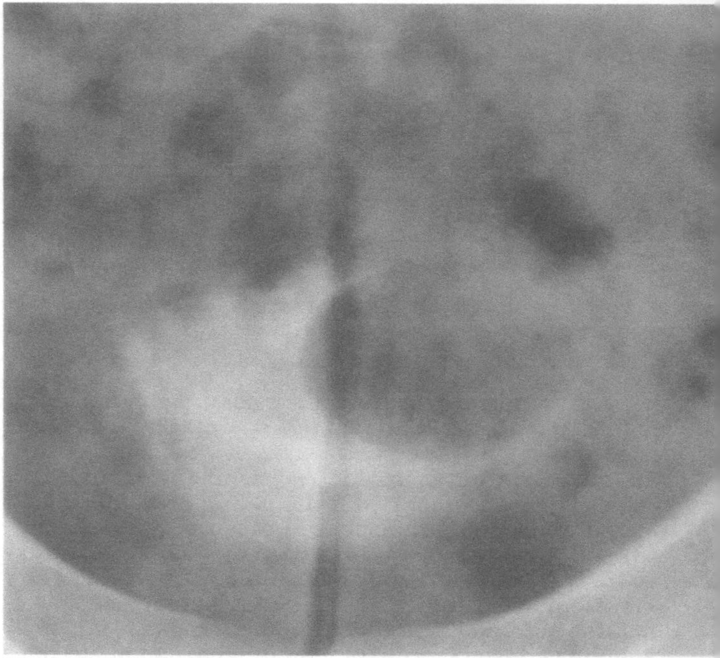

Figure 2.4. Ureterocoele. There is a large, round, filling defect in the bladder, due to the ureterocoele.

21

situation, posterior (Figure 2.2) or even medially pointing calyces. There will be a corresponding rotation of the pelviureteric junction and the more severe the rotation the more likelihood of pelviureteric obstruction and hydronephrosis. The diagnosis is usually made on the IVU, but in doubtful cases the isthmus can be shown on a radioisotope study, preferably an AP projection.

Duplication

Duplication can be unilateral or bilateral, and can vary from a bifid collecting system to a complete duplication

with separate insertion of the ureters (see Figure 2.3). When there are two separate ureters, the ureter draining the upper renal moiety invariably inserts caudally and may have an ectopic insertion. In extreme cases it can insert, for instance, into the vagina when there will be permanent incontinence. The upper moiety is more likely to be the site of infection and subject to hydronephrosis. There is an association between duplicity and ureterocoele when the 'filling defect' of the ureterocoele (Figure 2.4) obstructs the upper moiety of a duplex system causing hydronephrosis. Radioisotope studies will demonstrate the differential function in the two (or rarely three) moieties.

3. Infection

Acute Pyelonephritis

In most cases of acute pyelonephritis the IVU is not helpful, but there may be an increase in renal size, impaired function and attenuated calyces due to renal oedema. Linear streaking of the pelvis due to the oedema is occasionally seen (see Figure 3.1). This finding is also associated with long-standing reflux.

A dense nephrogram with a poorly developed pyelogram has occasionally been described, and is likely to be due to blockage of the ureter by pus. Nonobstructive hydronephrosis and acute pyelonephritis are recorded and are thought to be attributable to reduced ureteral peristalsis as a result of *Escherichia coli* endotoxins.

Pyeloureteritis Cystica

Pyeloureteritis cystica is characterized by the presence of small, translucent, round filling defects in the renal pelvis and ureter, and often occurs without any obvious cause although it is considered to be the result of

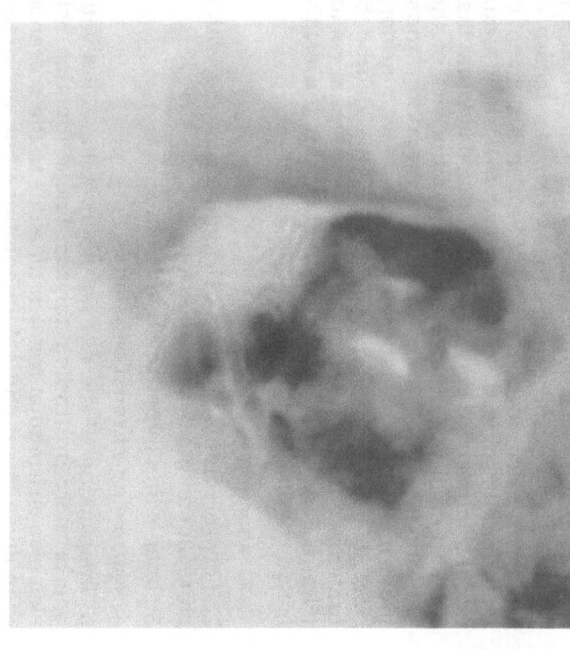

Figure 3.1. *Mucosal striations of the pelvis and major calyces of the right kidney. This appearance is due to oedema in acute pyelonephritis or recurrent reflux. In this case, there is acute pyelonephritis and the oedema has resulted in attenuation of the pelvicalyceal system.*

infection. A similar appearance is seen in schistosomiasis (see Figure 3.2).

Chronic Atrophic Pyelonephritis

Chronic atrophic pyelonephritis is a disease of childhood and is almost invariably accompanied by reflux. It is one of the commonest causes of renal failure in children. Vesicoureteric reflux is found in 90 per cent of children with scarred kidneys, and when ureteric reflux and intrarenal reflux are demonstrated, it is found that the site of backflow in the kidney is the site of the subsequent renal scarring. It is, therefore, most important when investigating children with urinary tract infections to assess accurately the degree of ureteric reflux and the presence of intrarenal reflux (Figure 3.3). The radiological features of the established condition (Figures 3.4 and 3.5) are:

1. A reduction in renal size.

2. Focal or multifocal areas of irregular scarring, with a corresponding calyceal deformity.

3. Intervening hypertrophied tissue.

4. Narrowing of renal substance.

5. Interruption of the normal interpapillary line with one or more protruding calyces. Foetal lobation will also give an irregular renal outline due to the presence of multiple sharp cortical indentations but, unlike the

Figure 3.2. *Ureteritis cystica in schistosomiasis in a male Egyptian patient with marked hydronephrosis from ureteral stricture. Retrograde study shows multiple translucent filling defects in the pelvis.*

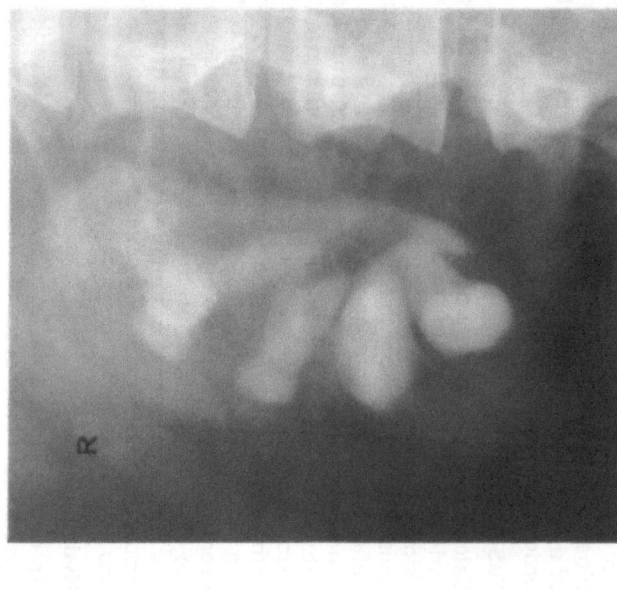

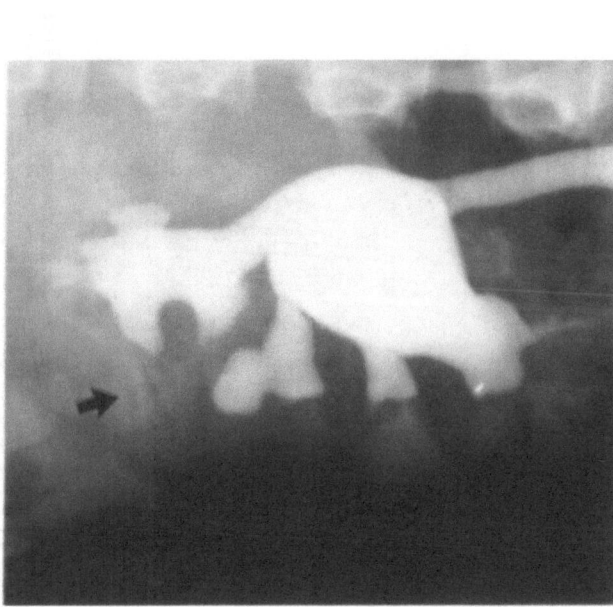

Figure 3.3. Intrarenal reflux in a female child with urinary tract infection. The micturating cystogram shows clubbed calyces, and linear streaks of contrast extending into the renal substance representing intrarenal reflux.

Figure 3.4. Bilateral chronic pyelonephritis (IVU). There is irregular cortical thinning, clubbing of the calyces and a coarse scar overlying a lower calyx. The interpapillary line is interrupted. Right kidney measures 10.4 cm.

scars of chronic atrophic pyelonephritis, which overly the normal calyces, the indentations alternate with calyces.

Normal kidneys are symmetrical, with less than 1.5 cm difference in length. A greater difference is suggestive of disease, and it is important to record the length in order that the disease can be monitored.

Tuberculosis

Calcification commonly occurs with tuberculosis and varies from a fine cloudy appearance to extensive calcification in tuberculous auto-nephrectomy. On the contrast examination the earliest change is loss of definition of a minor calyx which progresses, if the condition is untreated, to a cavity which communicates with deformed calyces (Figure 3.6). The inflammatory reaction leads to the narrowing of the infundibulum with eventual isolation of the tuberculous cavity, which can then progressively dilate. Scarring, similar to that seen in chronic focal pyelonephritis, will result and, if the disease continues, ureteric narrowing will eventually isolate the whole kidney and a pyonephrosis will result. With time, extensive calcification develops (Figure 3.7).

Hydatid Disease

An uncomplicated, isolated hydatid cyst is indistinguishable from other cysts, but if the walls are calcified the

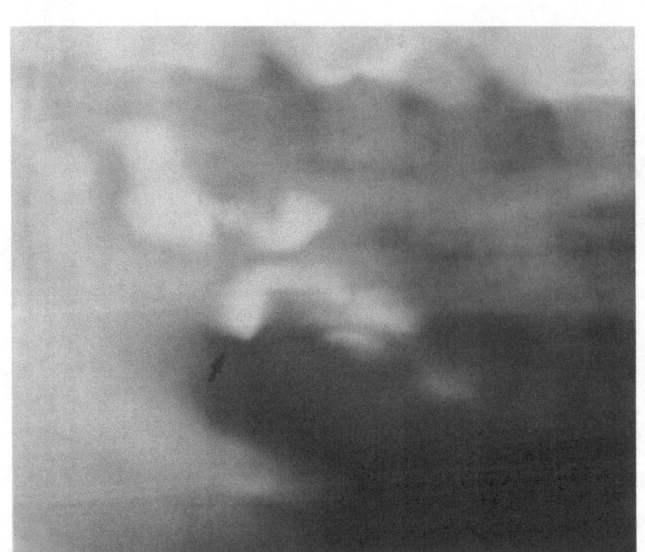

Figure 3.5. Chronic focal pyelonephritis (zonogram). Note the irregularity of the renal outline, coarse scarring (arrowed), calyceal clubbing and lower pole hypertrophy.

daughter cysts may be visible within the mother cysts.

If communication with the collecting system occurs, which will eventually happen if the condition remains untreated, the contrast will enter the cyst on both intravenous urography and retrograde studies. The daughter cysts can be seen as characteristic filling defects likened to a 'bunch of grapes'.

Calcification may or may not occur. If it does, it is a typical curvilinear configuration (Figure 3.8).

Schistosomiasis

Direct involvement by schistosomiasis initially affects the lower urinary tract, and gives rise to characteristic radiological appearances with bladder and ureteric calcification and ureteric strictures. The kidneys can also be secondarily involved by obstructive uropathy due to either ureteric strictures or secondary calculus disease.

Xanthogranulomatous Pyelonephritis

Xanthogranulomatous pyelonephritis results from prolonged urinary tract infection and is more common in women than men. In the majority of patients there is a renal mass, and characteristically there are areas of radiolucency due to the presence of 'foam cells' (Figure 3.9 a and b). Angiographically the appearances are often indistinguishable from a malignant circulation.

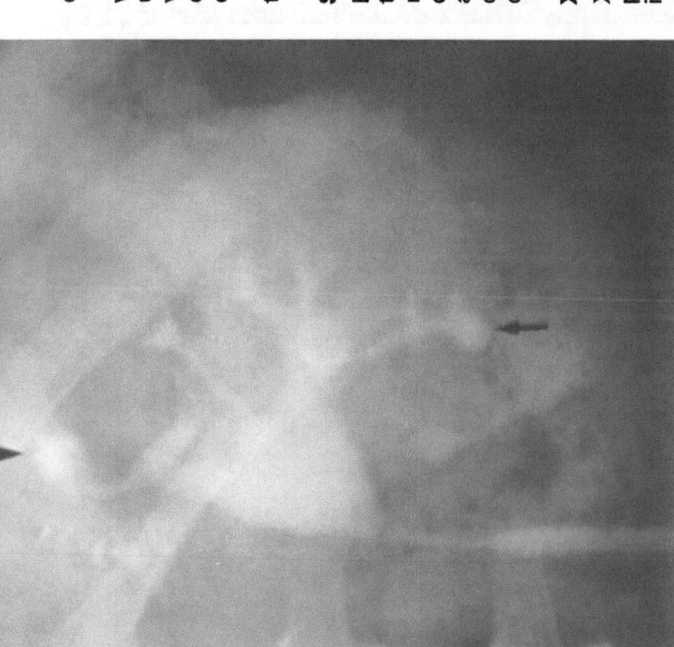

Figure 3.6. *Renal tuberculosis. Upper and lower pole tuberculous cavities (arrowed) communicating with deformed calyces. Note the narrowed infundibulum of the uppermost calyx. There is also upper medial calcification.*

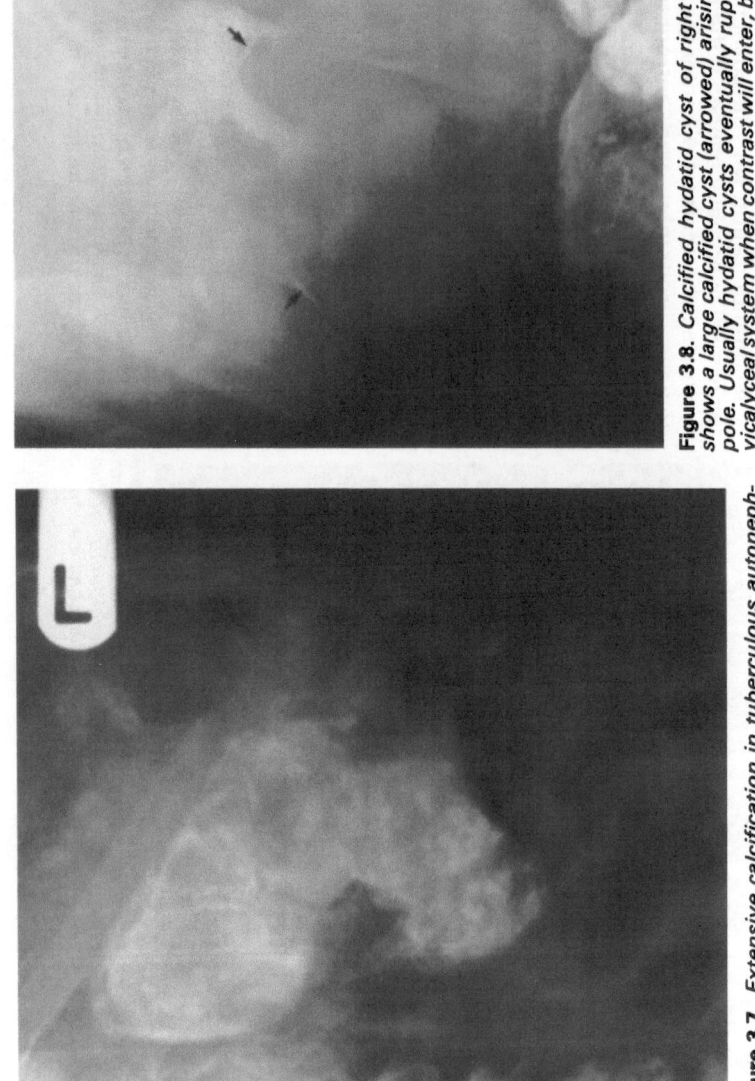

Figure 3.7. Extensive calcification in tuberculous autonephrectomy.

Figure 3.8. Calcified hydatid cyst of right kidney. IVU film shows a large calcified cyst (arrowed) arising from the lower pole. Usually hydatid cysts eventually rupture into the pelvicalyceal system when contrast will enter, but this has not yet occurred in this case.

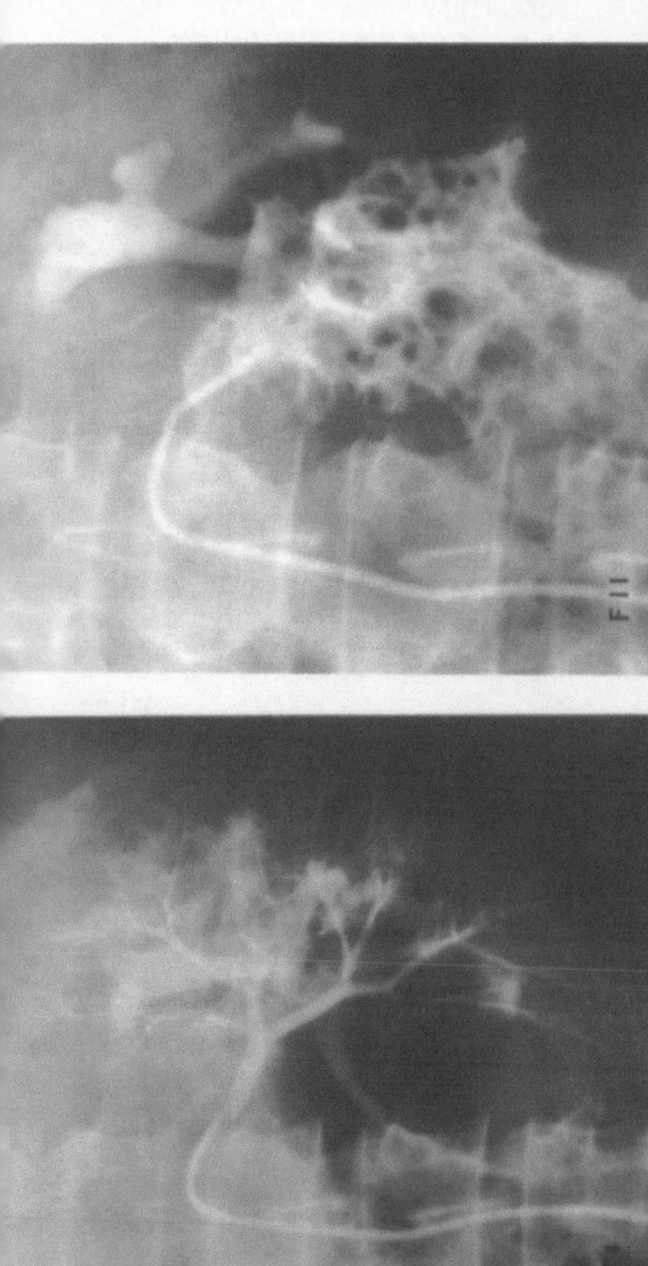

Figure 3.9. Xanthogranulomatous pyelonephritis in a female patient aged 17 years with a history of urinary tract infection. IVU showed a kidney 19 cm long with multiple parenchymal defects and diffuse deformity of calyces. The kidney had a dual arterial supply. **(a)** The arterial phase of a selective catheterization of the upper vessel. Note the stretched vessels in all areas, but in this case no 'neovascularity'. **(b)** The late phase of the lower vessel with the multiple filling defects due to collections of fat.

Pyonephrosis

This term, which means a distention of the pelvicalyceal system by pus, is normally taken to include acute and chronic pyonephrosis and infected hydronephrosis.

There is no characteristic radiological appearance, but a typical case would show the following features:

1. Plain film appearance: unilateral enlarged kidney with an ill-defined outline and psoas shadow. There would probably be calculus disease, in many cases a staghorn (see Figure 3.10).

2. High dose IVU: the kidney functions poorly but an irregular nephrogram can usually be achieved, often with 'rim sign' and 'crescents'. If a pyelogram is obtained there will be evidence of distention of the pelvicalyceal system, and an obstructing level may be confirmed.

3. CT scan: this would demonstrate the distended pelvicalyceal system and the attenuation factors would confirm the presence of pus. The loss of clarity between the dilated collecting system and the compressed parenchyma is a distinguishing feature from non-infected hydronephrosis, where there would be a clear line of demarcation.

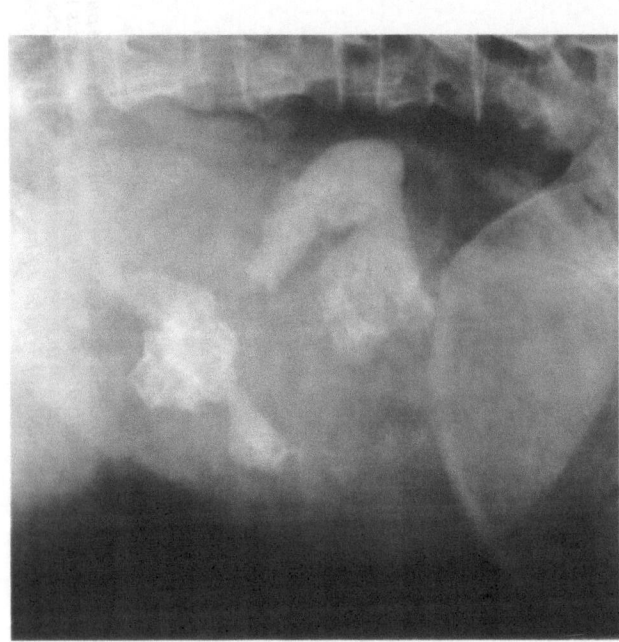

Figure 3.10. *Pyonephrosis associated with staghorn calculus. The kidney, which measured 18 cm, has enlarged 6 cm in five years. There was no function on IVU and at operation a pyonephrosis was found.*

ultrasonic criteria should be met:

1. The cyst should be well demarcated and echo free even with an increase in gain.
2. The wall should be smooth and well defined.
3. There should be a strong distal wall echo (Figure 4.1).

4. Investigation of Renal Masses

As mentioned in the introduction there are now sufficient sophisticated techniques available to allow a systematic approach to the investigation of renal masses in the shortest possible time and with minimal unpleasantness and hazard to the patient. Table 4.1 illustrates the investigative sequence that is widely followed when a mass is found on intravenous urography.

Ultrasound

Ultrasound, which is simple to perform, non-invasive, radiation free and independent of function is the first investigation and will indicate the consistency of the lesion.

Simple Cyst

A simple serous cyst may well be suspected as a result of nephrotomography (see below) but the following

Table 4.1. Investigation of renal mass.

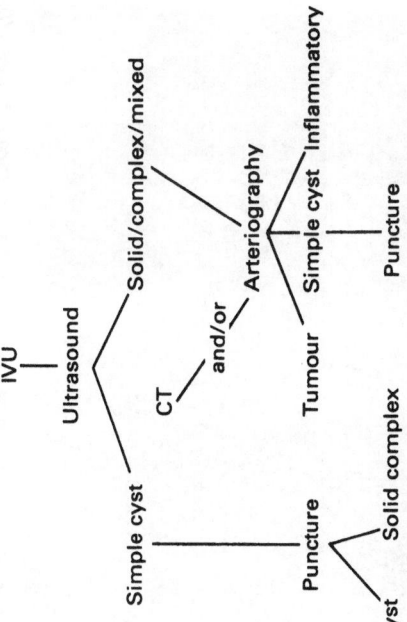

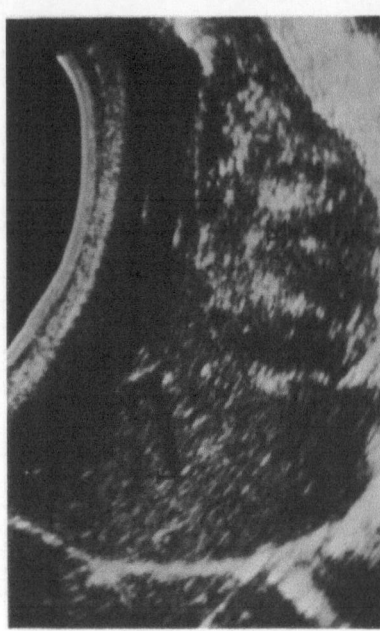

Figure 4.2. *Longitudinal ultrasound scan through liver (l), showing enlarged right kidney (k) with multiple irregular interfaces due to large hypernephroma replacing most of kidney.*

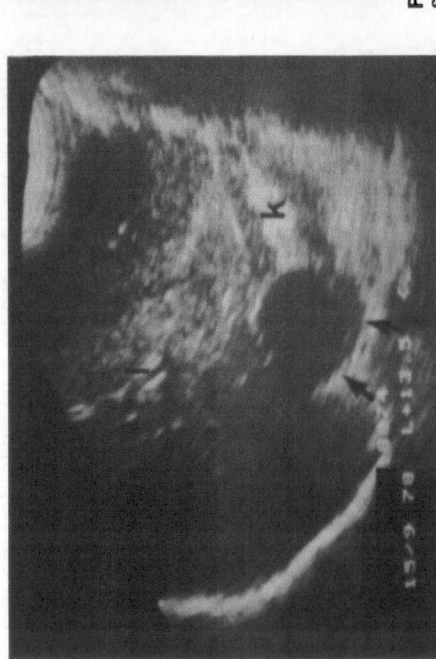

Figure 4.1. *Simple cyst of right kidney. Longitudinal ultrasound scan through liver showing a large cyst expanding the upper pole of the kidney. Note the enhanced posterior wall echo (arrows); k, kidney; l, liver.*

rate should be clear and free of cells and blood, and have a low urea and fat content.

Occasionally a solid tumour will be punctured, but there is considerable evidence that if this is the case there is little risk of spreading the tumour, and cytology can then be carried out.

Because a small percentage of cysts will have malignant cells within their walls ultrasonically guided cyst puncture should be carried out (Figure 1.8). The aspi-

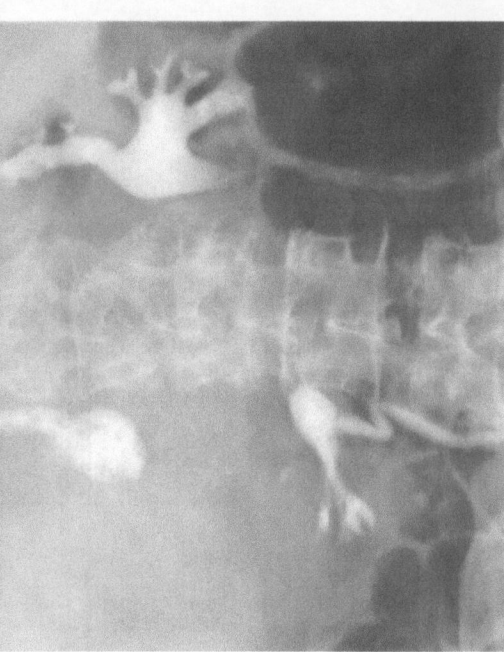

Figure 4.3. *Calcification in renal carcinoma. Large mass arising from the upper pole displacing the remaining renal tissue downwards. The upper calyces are directly involved and the lower calyces are displaced.*

Solid, Complex and Mixed Ultrasound Appearances

Solid lesions, which are usually due to vascular neoplasms, have wall echoes which are less well defined and smooth as the sound wave has been attenuated by multiple interfaces (Figure 4.2). The echo pattern of a solid tumour is usually greater than that of adjacent normal tissue but may be equal. Complex lesions show a basically cystic pattern, but with internal echoes, and may be due, for instance, to necrotic renal neoplasms, abscesses, infective cysts or occasional cases of hydronephrosis. The mixed lesions show cystic appearances in one area and complex echoes in another. Xanthogranulomatous pyelonephritis will give this pattern.

CT guided biopsy or arteriography is the next step depending on the facilities available.

Intravenous Urography

Plain Film

Expanding lesions may lead to a localized bulge on the renal outline or generalized enlargement, particularly with tumours and especially if the renal vein is involved.

The alignment of the kidney may be altered; for instance, an upper pole lesion will displace the kidney downwards (Figure 4.3). A normal variant which

should not be mistaken for a pathological mass is the so-called 'dromedary hump'. This is a bulge on the lateral border of the kidney which is almost always on the left side. In this condition the distance between the

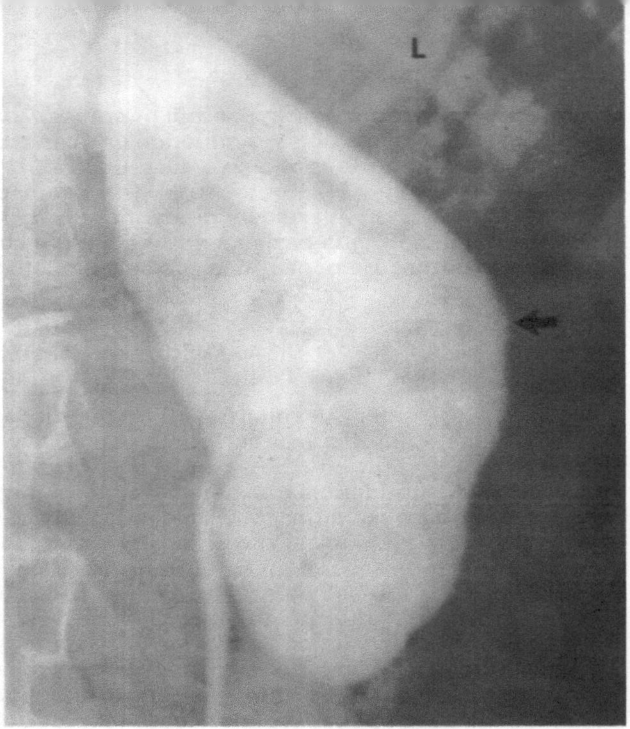

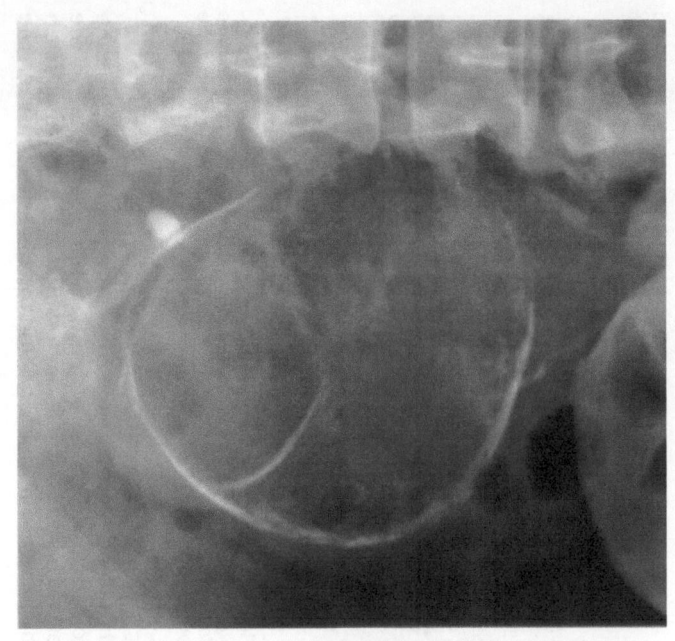

Figure 4.4. Normal dromedary hump on the left kidney (arrowed). An anterior hump is often seen on CT scans and, like the lateral dromedary hump, almost always affects the left kidney.

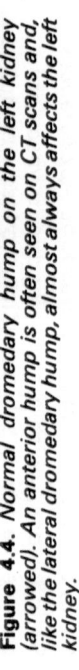

Figure 4.5. Curvilinear calcification in renal cyst. At operation a simple cyst was found.

renal margin and the underlying calyx is normal (Figure 4.4). Calcification occurs in six per cent of renal carcinomas (Figure 4.3) and three per cent of cysts (Figure 4.5). Typically, cystic calcification is linear or curvilinear while in a tumour it may take almost any form including curvilinear. Statistically, curvilinear calcification is more likely to be within a malignant neoplasm than within a cyst (Figure 4.6).

Nephrotomogram

Simple serous cysts will have a sharp cyst/parenchyma interface, a thin wall and, if projecting from the margin, may show the 'claw sign' (Figure 4.7).

Pyelogram

It is important to remember that if the lesion does not disturb either the pelvicalyceal system or the margin of the kidney it may well be missed. It is in this group that gamma camera studies are valuable.

Peripherally situated tumours may distort only a single calyx which will be stretched and elongated or appear clubbed, depending on the relationship of the lesion. More centrally placed lesions will involve multiple calyces with separation (see Figure 4.8). Calyceal amputation is unusual with simple cysts but often occurs with neoplasms. Likewise, simple cysts tend to give rise to simple types of calyceal deformity whereas malignant neoplasms lead to bizarre

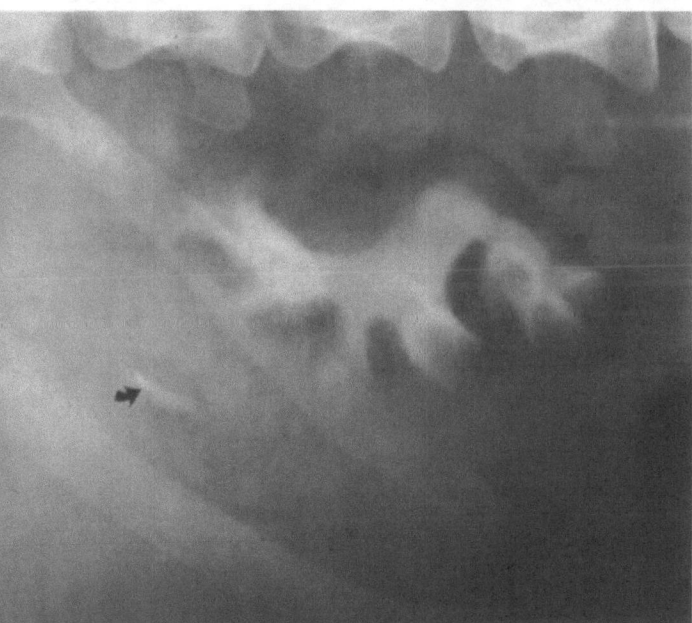

Figure 4.6. *Carcinoma of the upper pole of the right kidney. Note curvilinear calcification (arrowed) and early destruction of the upper calyces.*

35

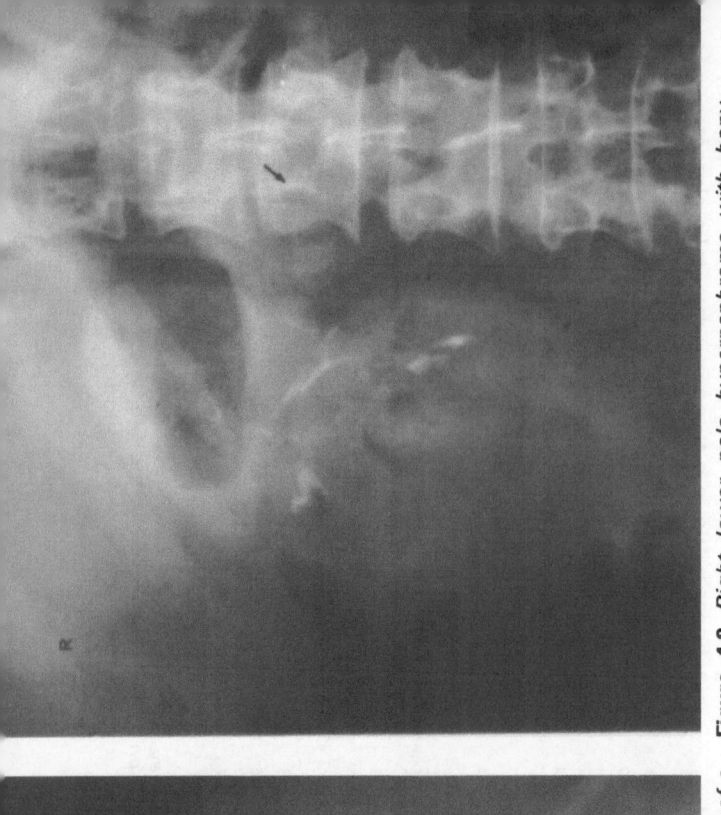

Figure 4.7. Nephrotomogram showing the 'claw sign' of a simple renal cyst. There is a well defined round lesion arising from the lower left renal pole. There is a clear demarcation from the normal tissue and the cyst is held by 'claws'. Note also the displaced calyces.

Figure 4.8. Right lower pole hypernephroma with bony metastases. Note the marked expansion of the lower pole (small arrows) and the splaying of the calyces. There is evidence of metastatic involvement of the transverse process, body and pedicle (large arrow) of the second lumbar vertebra.

appearances. If the pelvis is involved there may be displacement or a filling defect. Very large tumours can lead to a 'non-functioning kidney'.

Angiography

Simple Cyst

A simple cyst will cause vascular displacement but be avascular itself on the arterial phase. On the nephrogram phase there will be a translucent defect, often with a 'claw sign'. If the lesion is central, vessels may, of course, run across it.

Neoplasm

On the arterial phase a typical malignant circulation will be seen with multiple irregular beaded vessels, arteriovenous anastomoses, pools of contrast, early venous filling and anastomotic vessels (Figure 4.9). On the nephrogram phase the lesion will be of equal or greater density than the normal parenchyma and there may be blotchy areas of necrosis within it.

Differential Diagnosis

Other lesions which can give rise to neovascularity are hamartomata, xanthogranulomatous pyelonephritis and other inflammatory lesions such as a renal carbuncle (Figure 4.10).

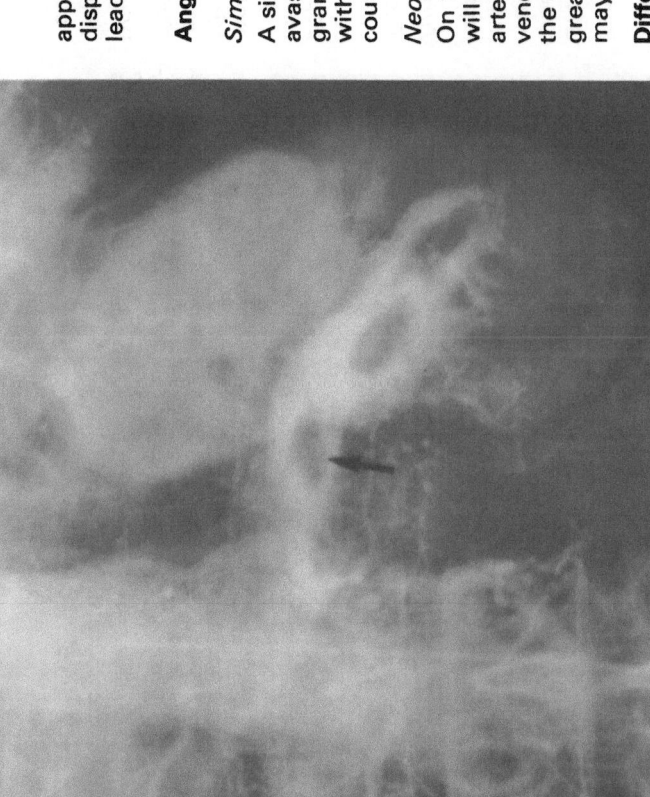

Figure 4.9. *Renal vein involvement by hypernephroma. On this mainstream arterial film there is early filling from a left lower pole hypernephroma with tumour spread to the vein shown as a filling defect.*

38

Other lesions that may be avascular include: papillary cystadenomata, invasive transitional cell carcinomas, lymphomas, metastases, an extensively necrotic tumour, infarcts and the less common benign tumours (Figure 4.11 a and b).

Renal Hamartomata

Of renal hamartomata, 40 per cent are associated with tuberous sclerosis and they may be unilateral or bilateral, solitary or multiple. On the plain film, lucent areas may be seen due to the presence of fat, and on arteriography characteristic corkscrew vessels occur.

Tumours of the Renal Pelvis and Ureter

The clinically important lesions of the renal pelvis and ureter are the transitional cell carcinoma and the squamous cell carcinoma. The former is usually a papilliferous lesion and may be multiple; the latter tends to be an ulcerating plaque.

The examination of choice is a high dose IVU with modifications if necessary, but a retrograde examination is not infrequently needed (Figure 4.12). If there is total obstruction, with hydronephrosis, an antegrade study may be required.

Wilm's Tumour

Wilm's tumour normally occurs in infancy and childhood but rarely in adolescence. There is usually a soft

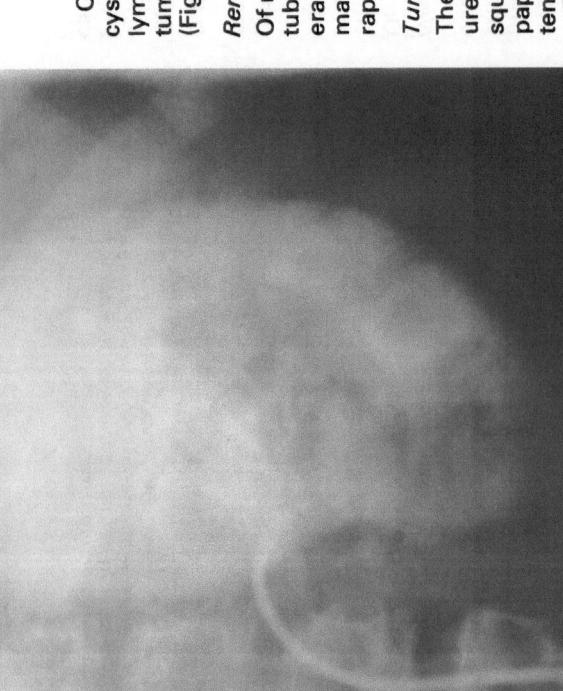

Figure 4.10. Renal carbuncle. A 13-year-old female was admitted with pyrexia, left loin pain, dysuria and vomiting. The IVU showed displacement of upper calyces and on the arterial phase of the arteriogram there was neovascularity. The nephrogram shows an expanded upper pole and vascular pooling. Despite the child's age, the lesion was thought to be a nephroblastoma, but histologically it proved to be a carbuncle.

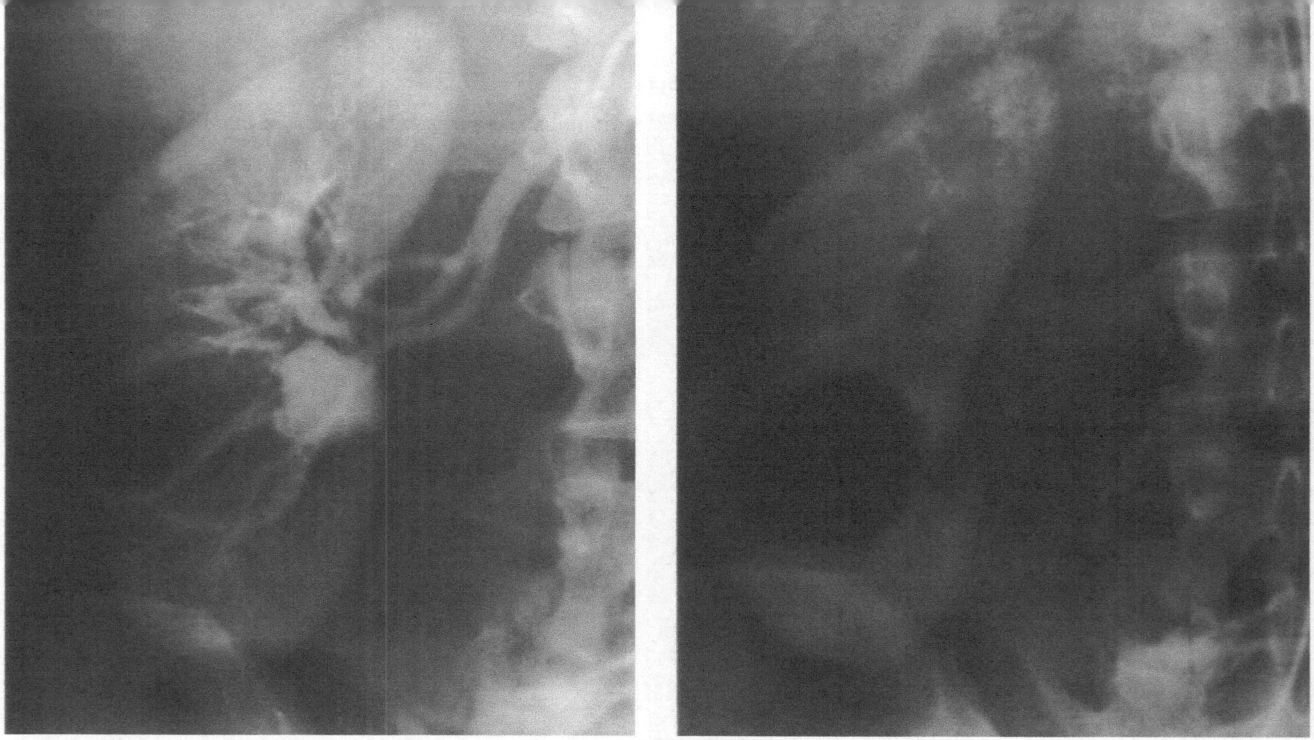

Figure 4.11. Renal adenoma in a 44-year-old female. (**a**) On the arterial phase of the selective angiogram there is vascular displacement but no malignant vessels. (**b**) On the nephrogram phase there is a lucent defect (arrowed).

39

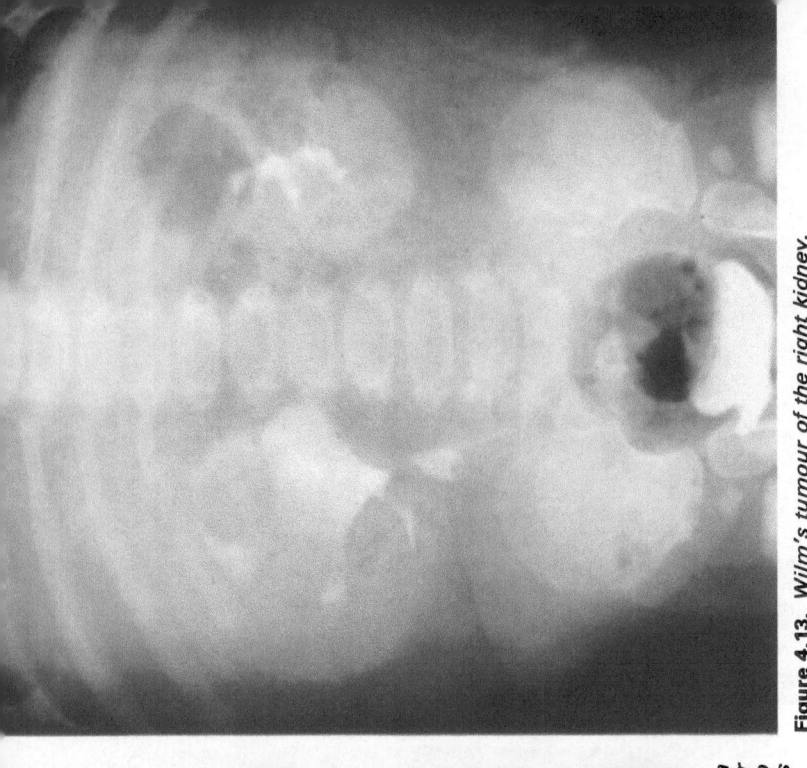

Figure 4.12 Transitional cell carcinoma of the renal pelvis in a male patient. Retrograde examination shows an irregular filling defect seen in the upper major calyx and extending to the minor calyces. Similar, but less definite, appearances were seen on the IVU.

Figure 4.13. Wilm's tumour of the right kidney.

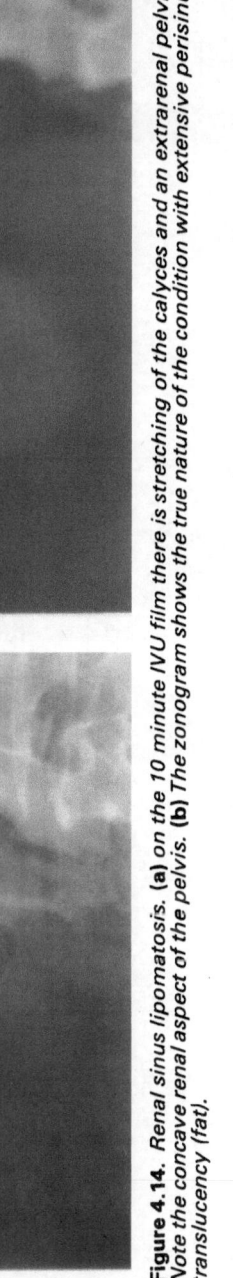

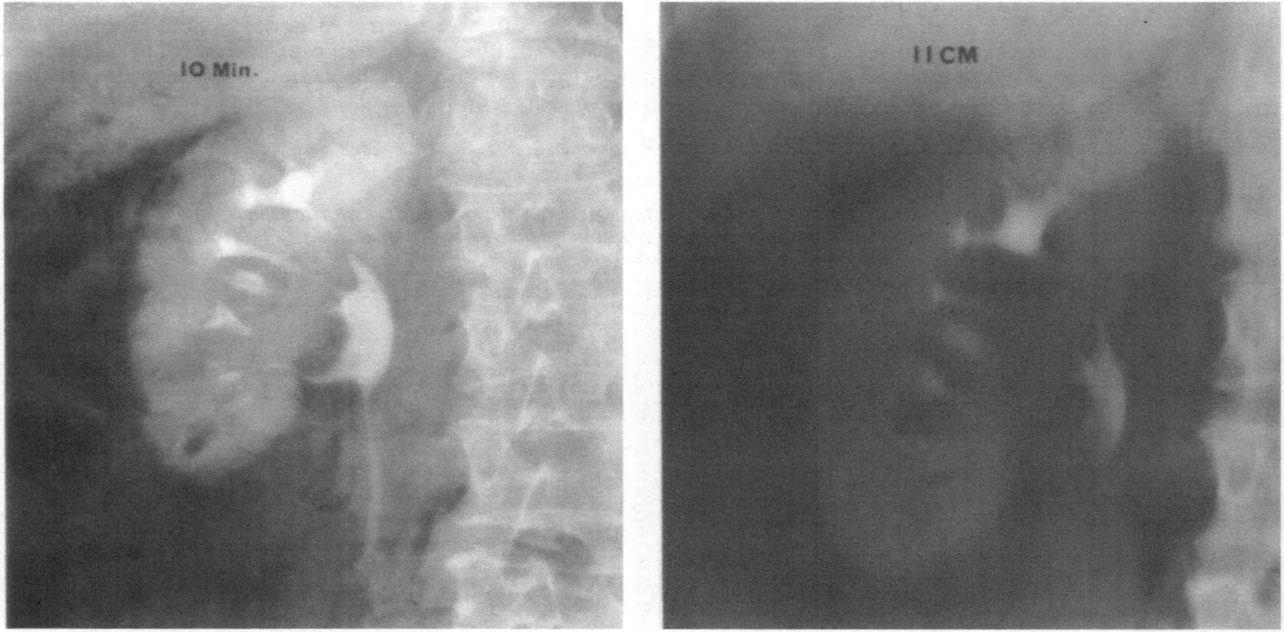

Figure 4.14. Renal sinus lipomatosis. (**a**) on the 10 minute IVU film there is stretching of the calyces and an extrarenal pelvis. Note the concave renal aspect of the pelvis. (**b**) The zonogram shows the true nature of the condition with extensive perisinus translucency (fat).

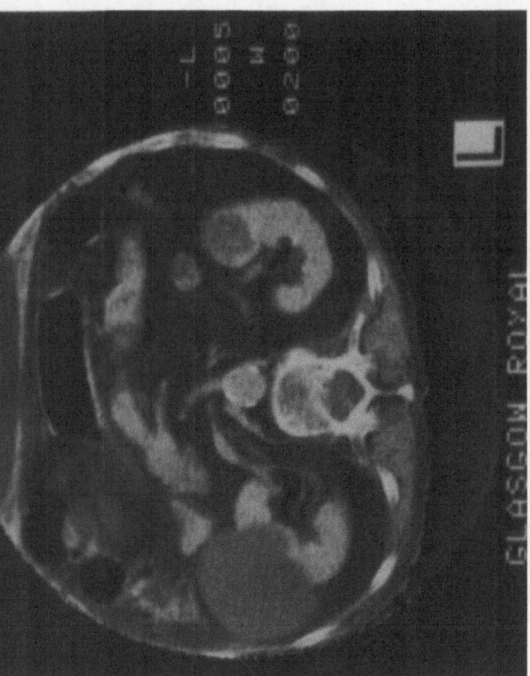

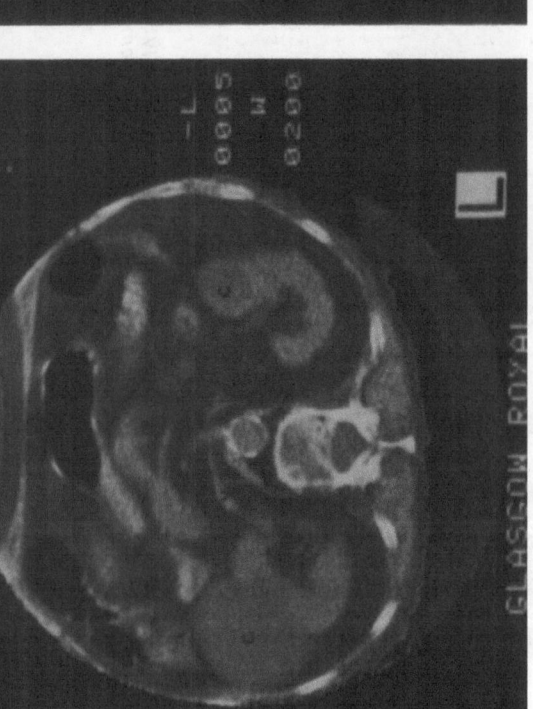

Figure 4.15. *Bilateral simple cysts.* **(a)** *On the initial scan there are two cysts, c, the attenuation values of which approximate water.* **(b)** *Following contrast enhancement, the renal substance increases in density but there is no change in that of the cysts, confirming their avascular nature. Inferior vena cava (v) draining renal veins.*

tissue mass displacing adjacent structures but calcification is rare and if there is function the IVU appearances are similar to a hypernephroma (Figure 4.13). If angiography is required there is usually, although not invariably, a rich neovascularity but arteriovenous malformations are not characteristic.

Metastatic Tumours to a Kidney

Unlike primary tumours, metastatic tumours do not have a characteristic small vessel circulation.

Pseudotumours

Ectopic islands of cortical tissue within the medulla

may present as space-occupying lesions displacing calyces on an IVU, but their true (benign) nature should be revealed on nephrotomography. Ultrasound is not helpful in the doubtful case as it will merely show a 'solid' lesion, but a DMSA study will show normally functioning tissue.

This variety of pseudotumour is common in the junctional zone between the upper and lower moieties of a duplex kidney.

Renal Sinus Lipomatosis

Well marked renal sinus lipomatosis can distort the pelvicalyceal system, so that on a plain IVU film a space-occupying lesion is suspected. However, tomography reveals the true nature of this benign condition (see Figure 4.14 a and b). Perisinus fat is also well shown on CT.

Computerized Tomography

Simple Cysts

The appearance of simple cysts is equivalent to that on the conventional nephrotomogram, and a 'claw sign' will often be seen (Figure 4.15 a and b). Simple cysts frequently appear as incidental findings on CT scans, and multiple cysts are found when only one was suspected. The attenuation factor of a cyst, which will be close to water density, will not alter with contrast enhancement.

Vascular Lesions

Following contrast injection there will be an increase in attenuation values. The lesion will have an attenuation value greater than or equal to that of a normal kidney. Involvement of the renal vein and inferior vena cava may be demonstrated.

5. Cystic Disease of the Kidney

The differential diagnosis and investigation of simple cysts has been described in the previous chapter. Three other cystic lesions of the kidney will be considered in this chapter.

Medullary Sponge Kidney

In this condition, which may involve a single papilla or the whole of both kidneys, the renal medulla is replaced by numerous small cysts. Unless secondary infection or calculus obstruction supervenes, renal function is normal, although if there is diffuse renal involvement the kidneys may be increased in size.

On the plain radiograph small calculi may be present, varying in number from a few to many hundreds, and these characteristically occur in groups. On contrast examination the cysts fill with contrast and they are characteristically round and smooth walled but may be

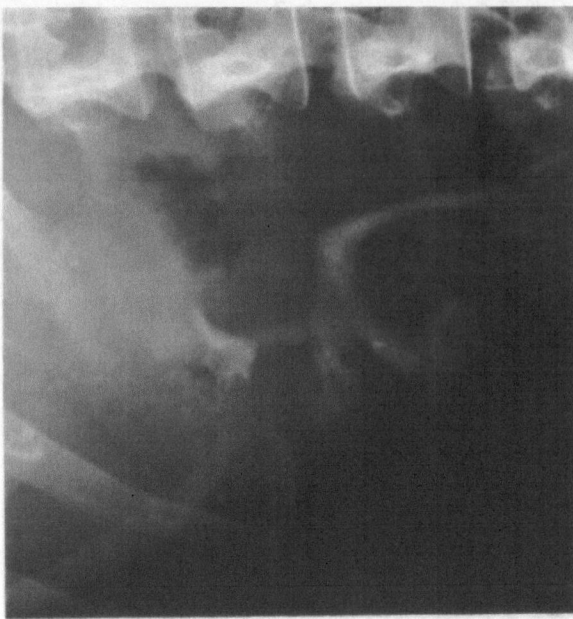

Figure 5.1. Medullary sponge kidney. On the plain films there were no calculi in this case. The IVU film shows multiple rounded cysts of varying sizes lying within the widened calyceal cups, and linear striations produced by contrast within dilated tubules.

irregular or linear shaped (Figure 5.1). The calyx maintains its normal shape with sharp marginal angles but the calyceal cup is increased to accommodate the cysts.

The differential diagnosis includes tuberculosis, well filled normal collecting systems and other forms of nephrocalcinosis.

Congenital Multicystic Disease

In congenital multicystic disease, which must be unilateral as the kidney is nonfunctioning, the normal renal substance is replaced by multiple cysts. It is the commonest cause of an abdominal mass in infancy and the most common cystic renal disease of infancy and childhood.

On the plain radiograph there may be a soft tissue mass, possibly with curvilinear calcification. The IVU will show nonfunction. The angiogram will show an absent or hypoplastic renal artery, and attempted retrograde examination will show a hypoplastic ureteric stump. Ultrasound and CT scanning will also confirm the presence of cysts.

Polycystic Disease

Polycystic disease of the kidneys exists in two forms: the infantile, which is invariably bilateral, and the familial adult form which is almost always, but not invariably, bilateral.

Adult Polycystic Disease

The adult form of polycystic disease normally presents in adult life with the onset of hypertension, renal failure, haematuria or renal colic, by which time the disease may have been transmitted to a subsequent generation. Of patients with polycystic disease, 80 per cent will give a positive family history. The disease may be more pronounced on one side than the other and result in different sized kidneys.

On the plain radiograph the renal outlines tend to be indistinct due to the lack of perirenal fat, but the kidneys are enlarged with a lobulated margin. On the IVU, if a pelvicalyceal system is preserved, the calyces and their infundibula will be elongated and stretched over cysts of varying sizes. A minor calyx in relation to a small adjacent cyst will be elongated but maintain its normal sharp margins (Figure 5.2). Seen end-on, bizarre appearances may be obtained with an apparent clubbing of calyces. If a major calyx is seen end-on stretched over a cyst, it may appear widened. Angiography is rarely needed except in patients with haematuria and suspected neoplasia, but if it is carried out the intrarenal vessels will be stretched over the adjacent cysts with an appearance not dissimilar to that

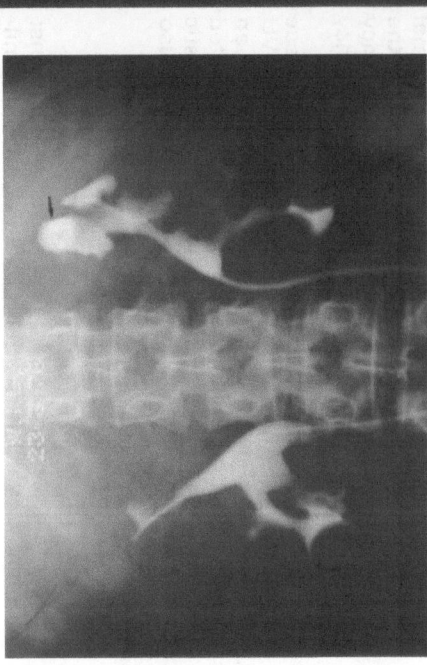

Figure 5.2. Polycystic kidneys, retrograde examination. Markedly enlarged kidneys with deformed calyces stretched over multiple cysts. Note how the minor calyces may be stretched over a cyst, resulting in an enlarged calyceal cup with normal sharp angles (curved arrow), or, if seen end-on, they may appear clubbed (straight arrow).

of hydronephrosis. However, in the latter condition the vessels have a more angulated appearance as compared to the vessels of polycystic disease. On the nephrogram the cysts will result in translucent defects

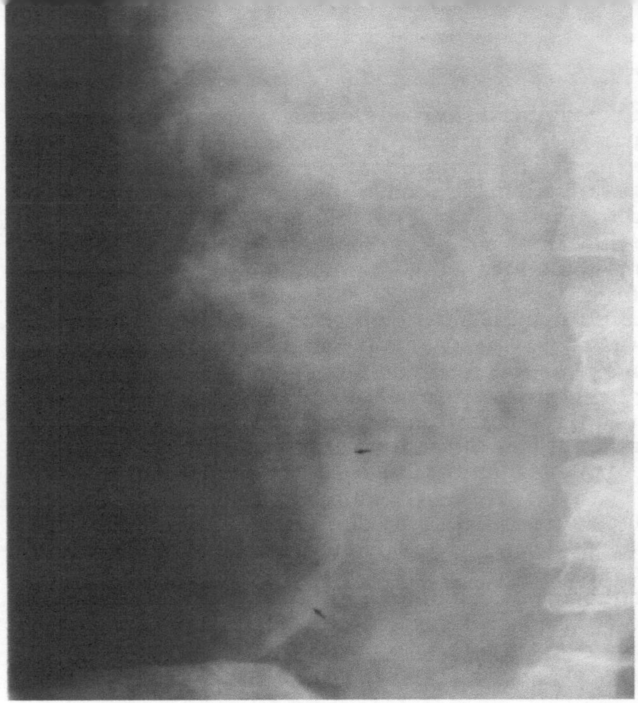

Figure 5.3. Polycystic kidneys. The five-minute film shows enlarged renal shadows with multiple rounded translucencies representing cysts. The functioning parenchyma is reduced to crescents surrounding the cysts and there is no normal pelvicalyceal system. A large lower right cyst is arrowed.

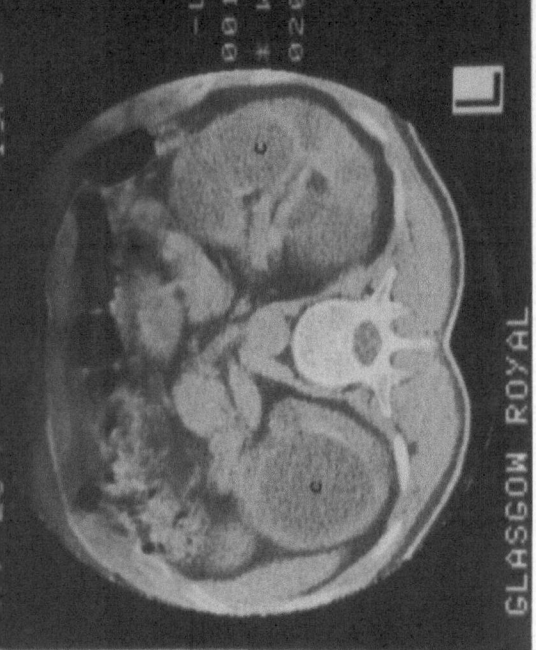

Figure 5.5. *Polycystic disease. The CT scan shows renal enlargement (the left kidney larger than the right) with multiple cysts, c.*

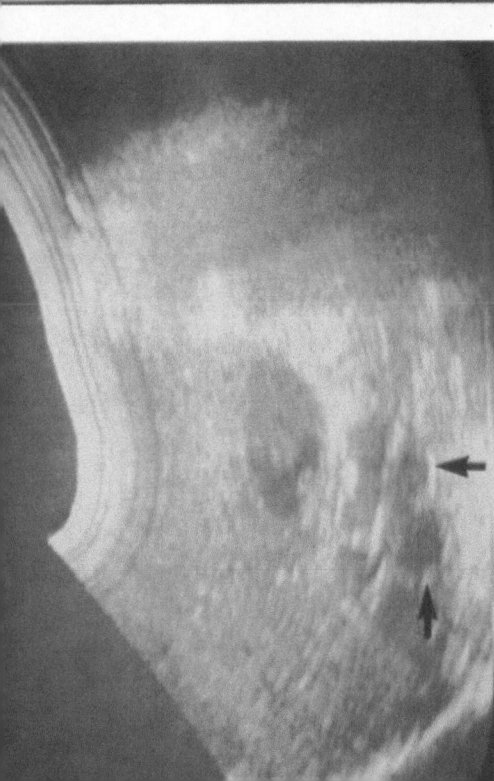

Figure 5.4. *Polycystic disease. Longitudinal ultrasound scan 6cm to the right of the midline through the liver. The right kidney is enlarged, lobulated and contains multiple cysts. Note the enhanced posterior wall echoes (↑) and the compressed parenchymal cresents (→).*

(Figure 5.3). In advanced disease there may be no pelvicalyceal system and merely multiple 'crescents' of compressed parenchyma. Calcification may be present, taking varied forms, not only curvilinear. The

appearances on ultrasound (see Figure 5.4) and CT scanning (see Figure 5.5) are characteristic. There is an association between renal polycystic disease and cystic disease of the liver.

47

6. Renal Failure

The principal aims of radiology in renal failure are:

1. To prove or disprove the presence of an obstruction.
2. To assess parenchymal disease.

The initial investigation is usually the high dose intravenous urogram.

The High Dose Intravenous Urogram in Renal Failure

Contraindications

There are now few contraindications, and high dose studies can be carried out even in the presence of oliguria or anuria. Myeloma was originally considered a contraindication, but since dehydration is not carried out in the presence of renal failure this no longer applies. Hepatorenal disease is a relative contraindication as the liver provides one of the main alternative pathways for the excretion of contrast, but if dialysis is available for treating possible allergic reactions the examination can still be performed.

In the presence of established or incipient cardiac failure the osmotic load, which will be dealt with slowly, might precipitate the patient into cardiac failure, and this should be carefully assessed.

Contrast Agents

Any of the standard contrast agents can be used in a dosage of approximately 2.2 ml per kg of urographin 60 or equivalent. As mentioned previously, there is evidence that better pelvicalyceal definition is obtained with the use of sodium rather than meglumine, though risks of giving a large sodium dose in renal failure must be considered.

Technique

Zonography is often required and preliminary cuts should be taken before the contrast injection is given to assess the optimum level. Delayed films may well be required if obstruction is present. Dialysis prior to the examination is helpful as it will stop the diuretic effect of uraemia. Table 6.1 shows the diagnostic 'sieve' in renal failure.

Further Examinations

If obstruction is shown to be present, antegrade and/or retrograde examinations may be necessary to clarify the site and nature of the obstructing lesion. Ultrasound, CT scanning and radioisotope studies are

Table 6.1. The IVU in renal failure.

```
                    ? Extra-renal obstruction
                    /                        \
                  Yes                         No
                   |                           |
    May show nature and site              Kidney size
                                          /          \
                                      Small          Large
                                   'End stage'    Define nature
```

all of considerable value in the diagnosis or exclusion of obstruction. Ultrasound can show a hydronephrotic kidney (see Figure 6.1) as can a CT scan which will also,

with serial sections, show the level and nature of a possible obstructing lesion (see Figure 7.7). Isotope studies have a part to play in the diagnosis and follow-up of obstruction, particularly in children.

The Nephrogram in Renal Failure

Kelsey Fry and Cattel (1972) have shown that careful observation of a nephrogram can give valuable information in renal failure. With a high dose and careful radiographic technique a nephrogram can nearly always be achieved, even in acute tubular necrosis when the density will be adequate for biopsy.

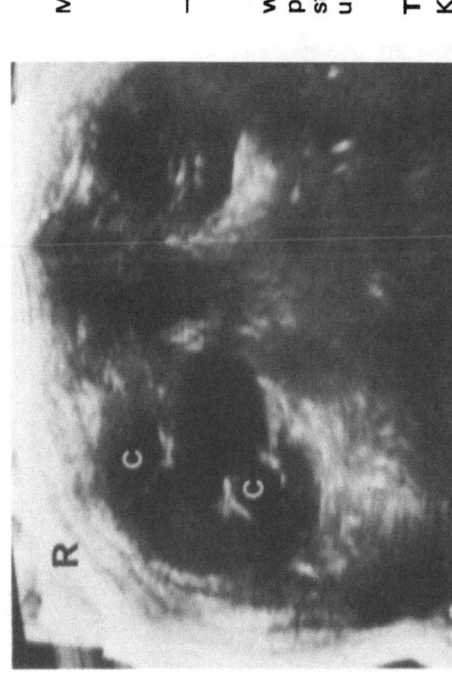

Figure 6.1. Right hydronephrosis. Ultrasound scan, transverse prone. The right kidney is enlarged with distended calyces adjoining the distended extrarenal pelvis. The transonic pelvicalyceal system is 'displacing' the compressed renal substance.

49

The authors describe three main groups of nephrogram:

1. The immediate faint persistent nephrogram.
2. The increasingly dense nephrogram.
3. The immediately dense persistent nephrogram.

The increasingly dense nephrogram occurs primarily in extrarenal obstruction, but also in 20 per cent of cases of acute tubular necrosis.

The immediate faint persistent nephrogram occurs when there is a reduction in the number of nephrons and glomerular filtration rate. This is maximal at the end of the injection and persists for a long time, although a reasonably good pyelogram is often obtained ultimately. The usual cause is chronic glomerular disease.

The immediate dense persistent nephrogram commonly occurs in acute tubular necrosis.

Plain Film Appearances

Apart from the size and shape of the kidneys, the presence or absence of calcification is an important diagnostic point. Calcinosis and calculi will be dealt with in chapter 7.

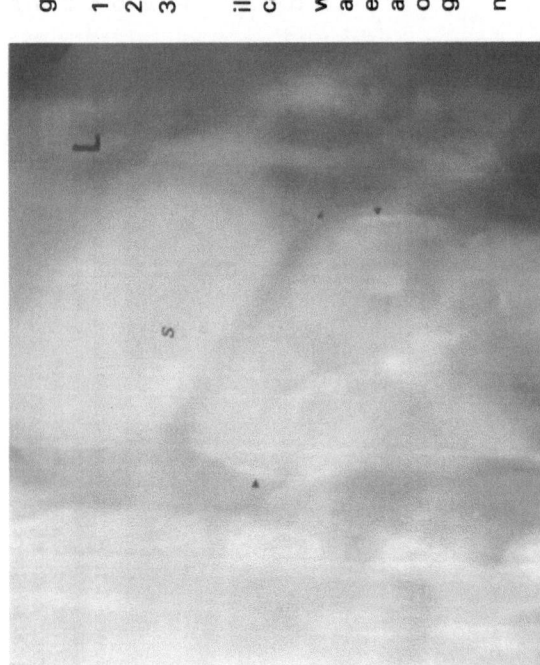

Figure 6.2. *Rim calcification in cortical necrosis. A 25-year-old female who survived acute cortical necrosis following antepartum haemorrhage. The kidney has a slightly irregular outline with a thin rim of cortical calcification (arrowed). Note the soft tissue density (s) above the kidney on this zonogram. This is the gastric fundus and should not be mistaken for a phaeochromocytoma.*

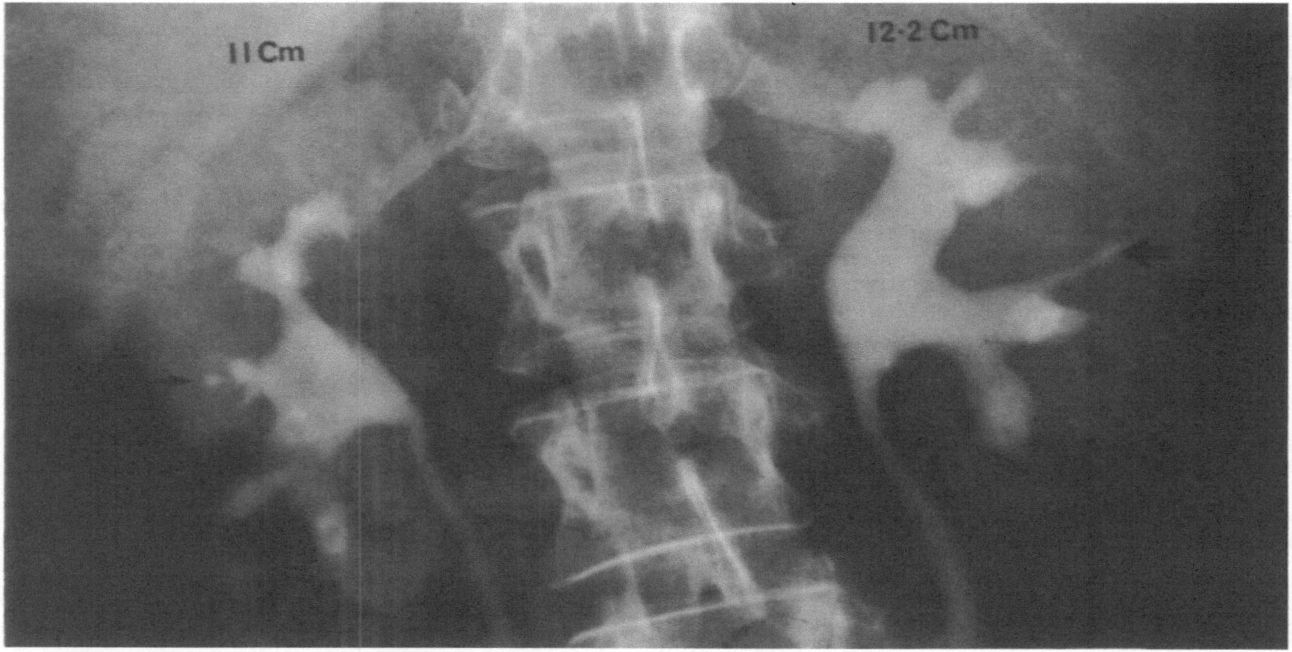

Figure 6.3a. Analgesic nephropathy in a female patient who was a known phenacetin taker. The initial film on a high-dose IVU shows normal sized kidneys with diffusely formed calyces, a central cavity (small arrow) and fistulous tracts (broad arrow).

results, with the calcified rim and calcification extending into the columns of Bertin, and this can occur in as little as 30 days.

Diffuse Parenchymal Calcification

Diffuse parenchymal calcification occurs rarely in patients with chronic glomerulonephritis or other long-standing renal disease.

Calcification in polycystic disease may occur in rings or curvilinear streaks, but may also be in the form of small flecks or irregular amorphous calcification.

Bilateral Small Kidneys

Bilateral small kidneys represent the irreversible stage of chronic renal disease and may be due to a number of factors, commonly arterionephrosclerosis, chronic glomerulonephritis, bilateral ischaemia or chronic pyelonephritis. Other causes include postobstructive atrophy (bilateral), late cortical necrosis, gouty nephritis, the collagen diseases, Kimmelstiel–Wilson disease and chronic interstitial nephritis.

The margin of the kidney is a most important diagnostic point. If it is scarred and irregular with areas of hypertrophy, chronic pyelonephritis or possibly multiple infarcts are the most likely cause. In chronic pyelonephritis the calyces will be deformed.

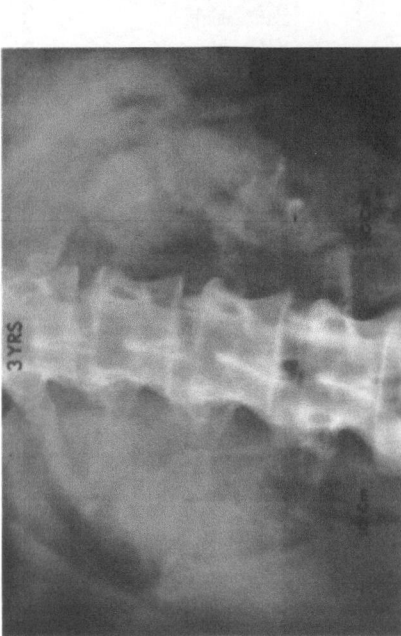

Figure 6.3b. *Same patient as Figure 6.3a, three years later. The kidneys have shrunk and the papillae calcified. Note the characteristic calculus with central lucency due to the sloughed papillae. The kidneys are now scarred.*

Cortical Calcification

In cortical calcification there is a thin rim of peripheral calcification (see Figure 6.2), and the usual cause is renal cortical necrosis due to a complication of pregnancy. If the patient survives a shortened kidney

If the renal outlines are smooth, chronic glomerulonephritis or chronic nephrosclerosis are the most likely causes but in the latter condition there is likely to be some surface irregularity from small infarcts. Bilateral renal artery stenosis also leads to bilateral smooth kidneys. In infarction the calyces tend to be normal apart from some minor distortion due to fibrosis.

Although bilateral shrunken kidneys in the presence of uraemia represent the 'end stage kidney' it is most important that any additional obstruction which is treatable should be excluded.

A condition which is frequently confused with chronic pyelonephritis is advanced analgesic nephropathy.

Analgesic Nephropathy

Analgesic nephropathy is one of the causes of papillary necrosis along with diabetes, obstruction, pyelonephritis and sickle cell anaemia but nowadays it is the most common one.

The condition is included in this section because although in early cases the renal size is normal, with advanced disease there is global shrinkage and an irregular wavy border (Figure 6.3 a and b).

Early in the disease when there is only papillary swelling there may be no obvious radiological change or, at the most, slight widening of the calyceal cup. Once necrosis develops, a fistulous tract can be seen extending out from the calyceal fornices (see Figure 6.3a), and if there is more extensive necrosis a cavity will be formed.

The tip of the papilla may be ultimately sloughed, giving rise to a triangular lucent filling defect (see Figure 6.3b). If it passes into the ureter and impacts, there will be evidence of an obstructive uropathy and the patient may be precipitated into acute on chronic renal failure.

An important differential point from chronic pyelonephritis is that in the latter condition there is good renal function on the IVU, even in advanced disease, whereas function tends to be reduced early in analgesic nephropathy. The age groups are also different, chronic pyelonephritis being a disease of childhood while analgesic nephropathy occurs in middle age.

In postobstructive renal atrophy there will be reduced renal function but the kidney will have a smooth outline and clubbed calyces.

Amyloidosis

It has recently been shown that in chronic amyloidosis, for example with rheumatoid arthritis, the kidneys are reduced in size (see Figure 6.4).

Bilateral Large Kidneys

The causes of bilateral large kidneys are bilateral obstruction, acute glomerulonephritis, acute pyelonephritis, acute tubular necrosis or cortical necrosis, polycystic disease, infiltration by lymphoma, leukaemia and myeloma, acute amyloid, and bilateral acute renal vein thrombosis. Infiltration by lymphoma, leukaemia and myeloma leads to enlarged kidneys with poorly visualized, stretched, collecting systems (Figure 6.5).

Arteriography and Renal Failure

There is a general vascular pattern which occurs in renal failure, with a reduction in the cortical blood flow and diversion through the juxtamedullary units. As a result, the density of the renal cortex is reduced and there is also a homogeneous nephrogram with the normal corticomedullary line of separation obliterated. The velocity of flow through the kidney will be reduced. The extrarenal arterial arcade is often demonstrated with greater ease and in greater detail than in the normal kidney.

Cardiovascular System and Uraemia

The chest radiograph may demonstrate evidence of cardiomegaly and cardiac failure, which will be

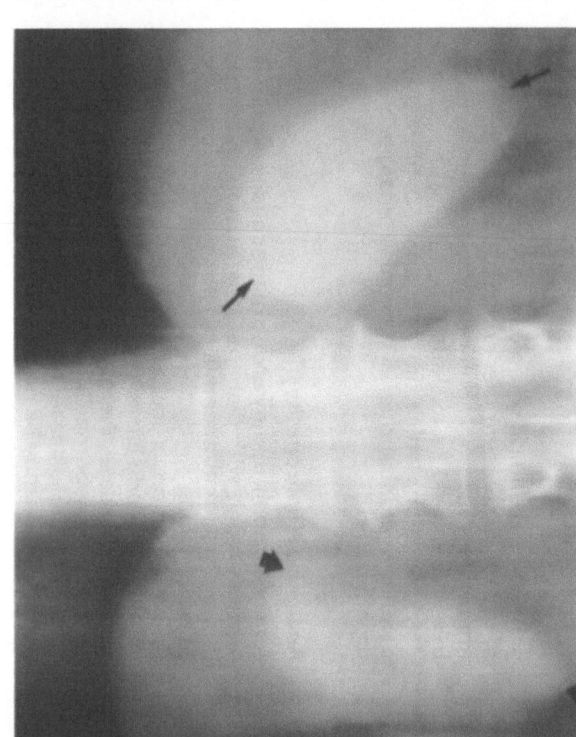

Figure 6.4. This 70-year-old female has had rheumatoid arthritis for many years and is now in renal failure. There is very poor function by both kidneys, which are small (10 cm) and have a smooth margin. The calyces are not well seen but are obviously not markedly distended. At post mortem amyloid was confirmed.

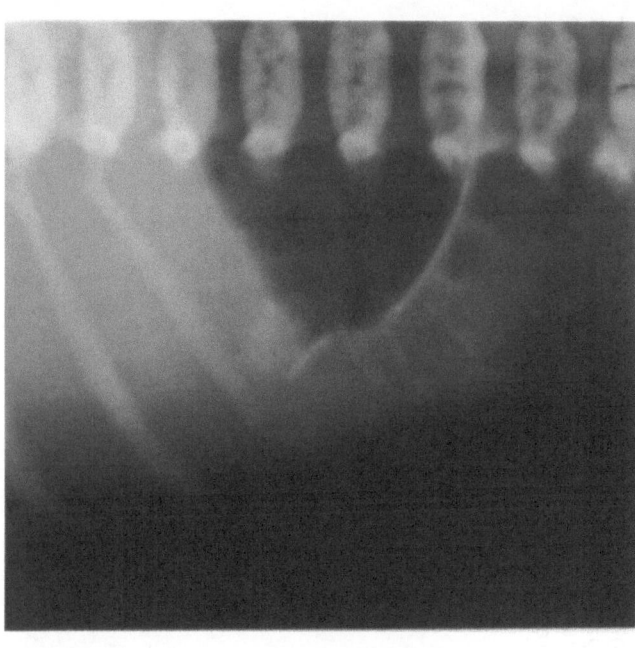

Figure 6.6. *Calcified renal vein thrombosis in an eight-day-old male following severe dehydration. It was confirmed at post mortem.*

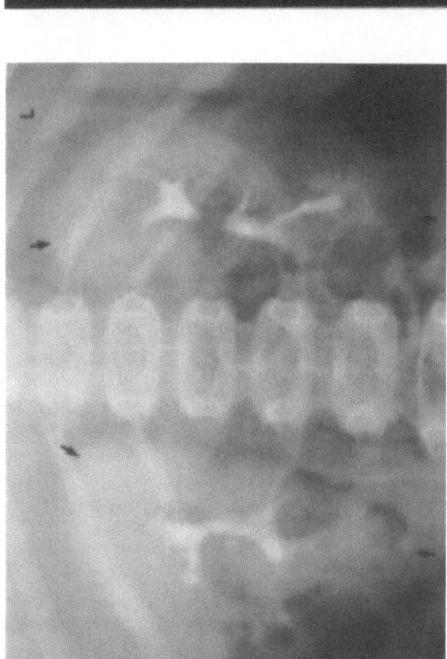

Figure 6.5. *Leukaemic infiltration of the kidneys. Note the diffuse enlargement of both kidneys (right = 10.5 cm, left = 11.0 cm), stretching of the pelvicalyceal systems and splenomegaly.*

dramatically affected by dialysis. Pulmonary oedema may be due to left-sided cardiac failure or possibly 'the uraemic lung'. Pericarditis may occur, and if a patient with an enlarged heart and ascites shows a reduction in response to dialysis, pericarditis is a likely cause.

Normal Sized Kidneys—Nephrotic Syndrome

In the active phase of the nephrotic syndrome the kidney size may be normal. On the IVU there will be a normal collecting system apart from slight infundibular stretching due to oedema. Pleural and peritoneal fluid is common and the pleural fluid usually collects in a subpulmonary situation.

The nephrotic syndrome has been considered to be a complication of renal vein thrombosis, but it is likely that there is nearly always underlying renal disease causing the thrombosis, particularly membranous glomerulonephritis. Renal venography is the investigation of choice in renal vein thrombosis. If a patient survives renal vein thrombosis, calcification in the renal veins may occur (Figure 6.6).

7. Nephrocalcinosis and Calculus Disease

Nephrocalcinosis

Nephrocalcinosis results from the diffuse deposition of calcium within the renal substance, in the form of multiple small rounded opacities and, less frequently, spicules of calcium. The causes fall into two main groups:

1. Hypercalcaemia or hypercalciuria.

2. The presence of biochemical or structural changes which favour the deposition of the calcium.

The main causes in group one are hyperparathyroidism, renal tubular acidosis (Figure 7.1), idiopathic hypercalciuria, sarcoidosis, multiple myeloma, carcinomatosis, Cushing's disease, steroid therapy, milk alkali syndrome and hypervitaminosis D. In group two: medullary sponge kidney, renal medullary necrosis and excessive intake of alkalis.

If nephrocalcinosis is associated with a staghorn calculus the likely causes are either renal tubular acidosis

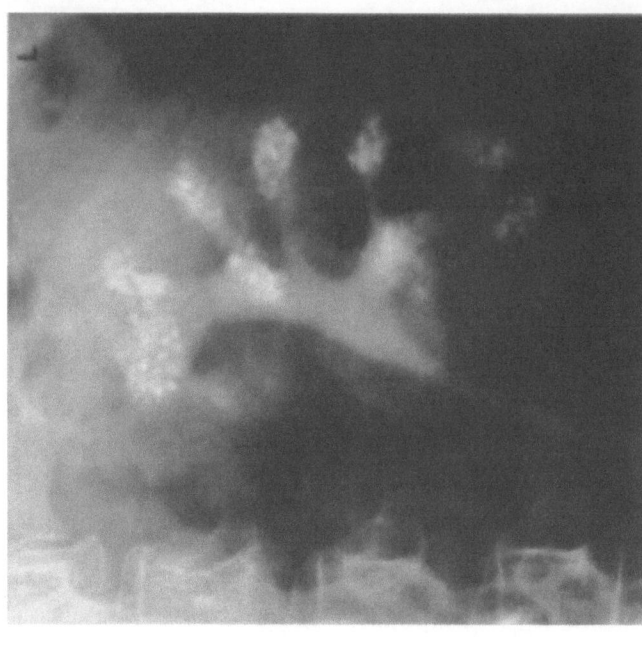

Figure 7.1. *Nephrocalcinosis in a female patient with known renal tubular acidosis.*

58

or idiopathic hypercalciuria. Renal tubular acidosis typically gives extensive dense calcification (Figure 7.1).

Conditions causing hypercalcaemia result in renal damage and reduction in renal size and include hyperparathyroidism, sarcoidosis and Cushing's disease. In this situation the calcinosis is slight to moderate. On the other hand, conditions which lead to hypercalciuria without hypercalcaemia, which include renal tubular acidosis and idiopathic hypercalciuria, will lead to a moderate or marked calcinosis with normal or increased kidney size.

In children, cretinism, hypophosphatasia and sulphonamide toxicity are likely causes.

Calculi

Causes of renal calculus disease are complex but there are certain predisposing factors such as metabolic disorders (for example hyperparathyroidism), structural abnormalities (for example pelviureteric obstruction and horseshoe kidneys) and, important in the tropics, dehydration.

Approximately 80 per cent of renal calculi are opaque and consist of calcium oxalate, phosphate or carbonate together with ammonium magnesium phosphate and urate stones (Figure 7.2). Cystine stones (Figure 7.3) are partly radio-opaque, and completely radiolucent cal-

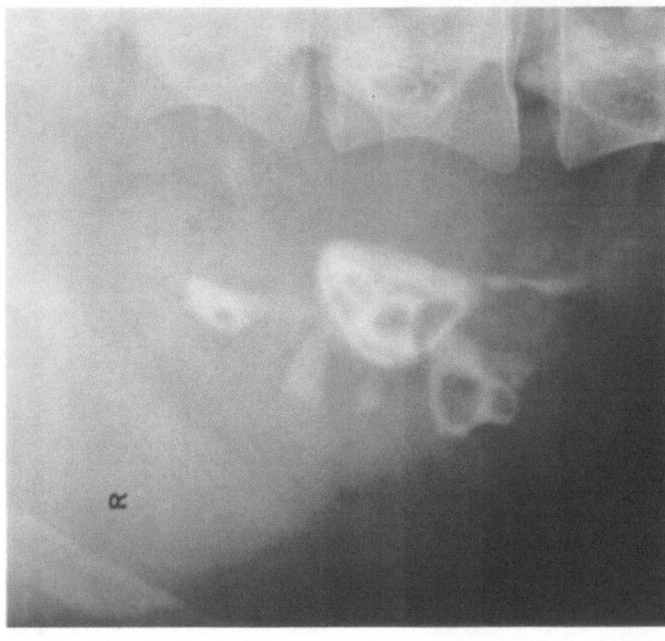

Figure 7.2. *Multiple translucent uric acid stones.*

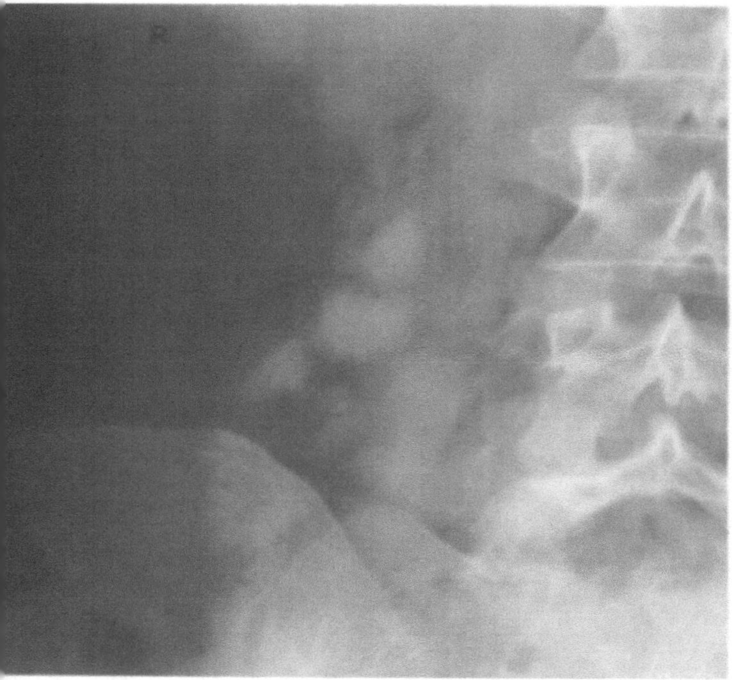

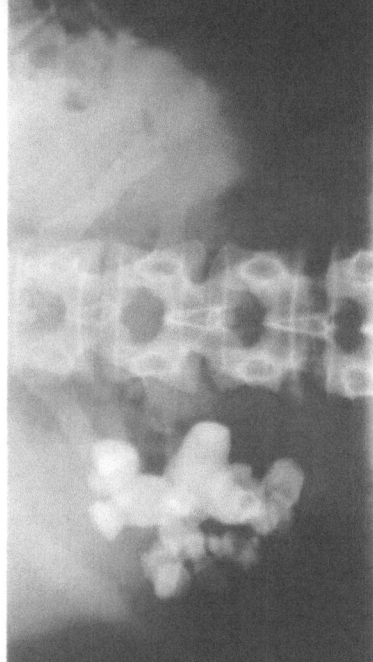

Figure 7.4. Staghorn calculus forming cast of the kidney.

Figure 7.3. Cystine calculi in the right kidney.

culi consist of pure uric acid, xanthine and the so-called 'matrix calculi'. The phosphate stones often grow very rapidly and can form a complete cast of the pelvis and calyces—a staghorn calculus (Figure 7.4). If the stones lie free within hydronephrotic cavities they will change their relationships with position (Figure 7.5 a and b).

Translucent calculi have to be distinguished from other lucent filling defects, the common causes of which are air, following a retrograde study or

59

60

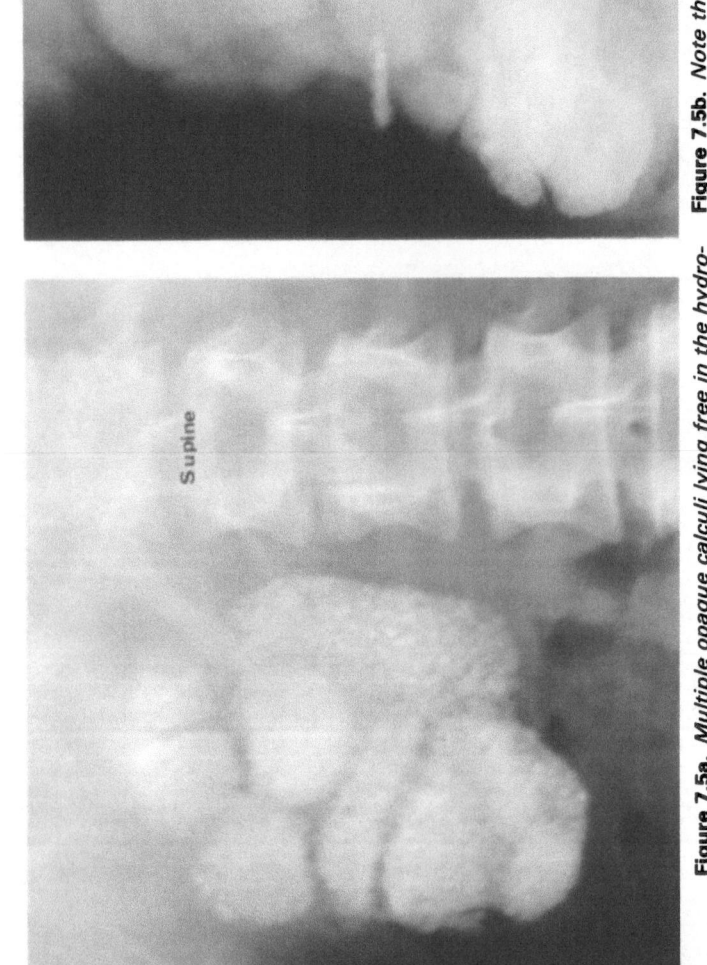

Figure 7.5a. Multiple opaque calculi lying free in the hydro-nephrotic kidney; patient in supine position.

Figure 7.5b. Note the levelling with the patient in the erect position.

vesicovaginal fistulae, blood clot (see Figure 7.6), pyelitis cystica, neoplasms and sloughed papillae. Non-opaque calculi may present on ultrasound as an echogenic structure with shadowing.

Acute Obstructive Uropathy

In acute obstructive uropathy there will be a progressive dense nephrogram with a delayed pyelogram. It may be necessary to take delayed films up to 24 hours to achieve the latter. If a pyelogram is obtained there will be clubbing of the calyces and a columnized ureter with moderate renal enlargement. In practice it is common for only the calyces to be filled with contrast, which layers below the urine in the dependent pelvic calyceal system (see Figure 7.7), and it is necessary to turn the patient prone in order to fill the ureter. It is essential to delay taking the prone radiograph(s) until the contrast has had time to diffuse down the ureter to the point of obstruction.

In acute obstruction there may be forniceal leaking with extravasation of contrast material. Although calculus obstruction is the commonest cause of peripelvic extravasation (see Figure 7.8), other causes are overenthusiastic compression, retrograde pyelography, trauma, polycystic disease, ureteral neoplasms or strictures, and tumours of the renal pelvis.

If angiography is carried out in acute obstruction there will be a prolonged transit time, and a slight

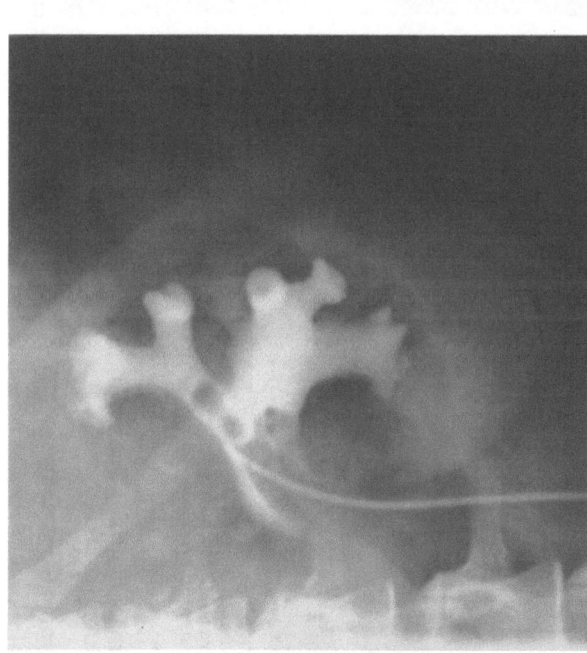

Figure 7.6. Blood clot in the renal pelvis in an 18-year-old male with severe haematuria. IVU showed a large, poorly functioning kidney. This retrograde film shows a blood clot in the renal pelvis and upper major calyx. Subsequent arteriogram showed traumatic arteriovenous aneurysms.

61

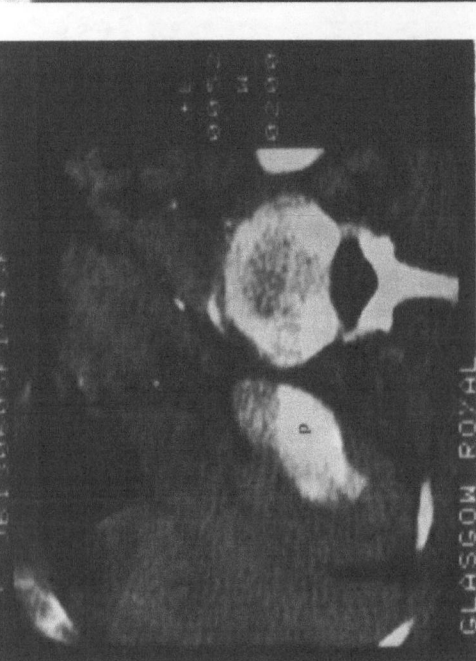

Figure 7.7. Hydroureter. CT scan shows contrast layering in a dilated extrarenal pelvis (p) in a case of obstruction; k, kidney; l, liver. The calcified opacities anterior to the vertebral body are osteophytes and calcification in vessels.

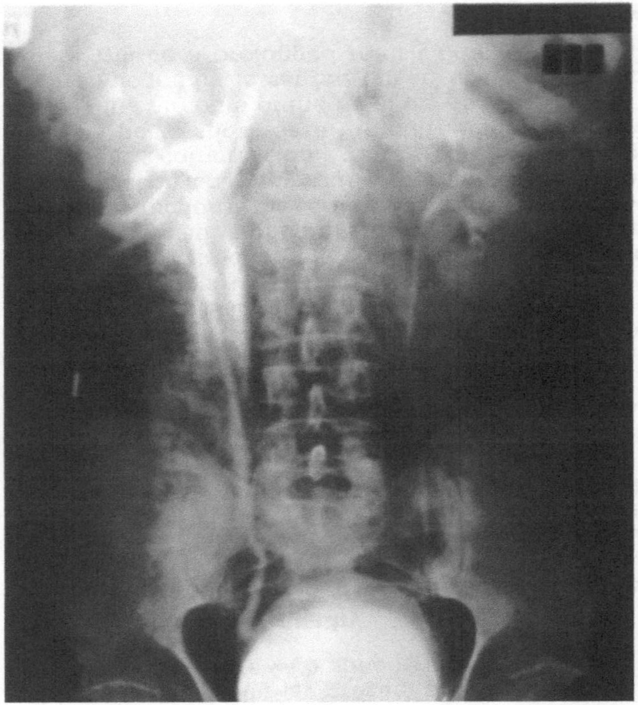

Figure 7.8. 'Spontaneous' rupture of the kidney with extensive extravasation of contrast.

spread of the intrarenal arteries with poor filling of spidery veins.

Chronic Obstruction

Prolonged obstruction results in marked dilatation of

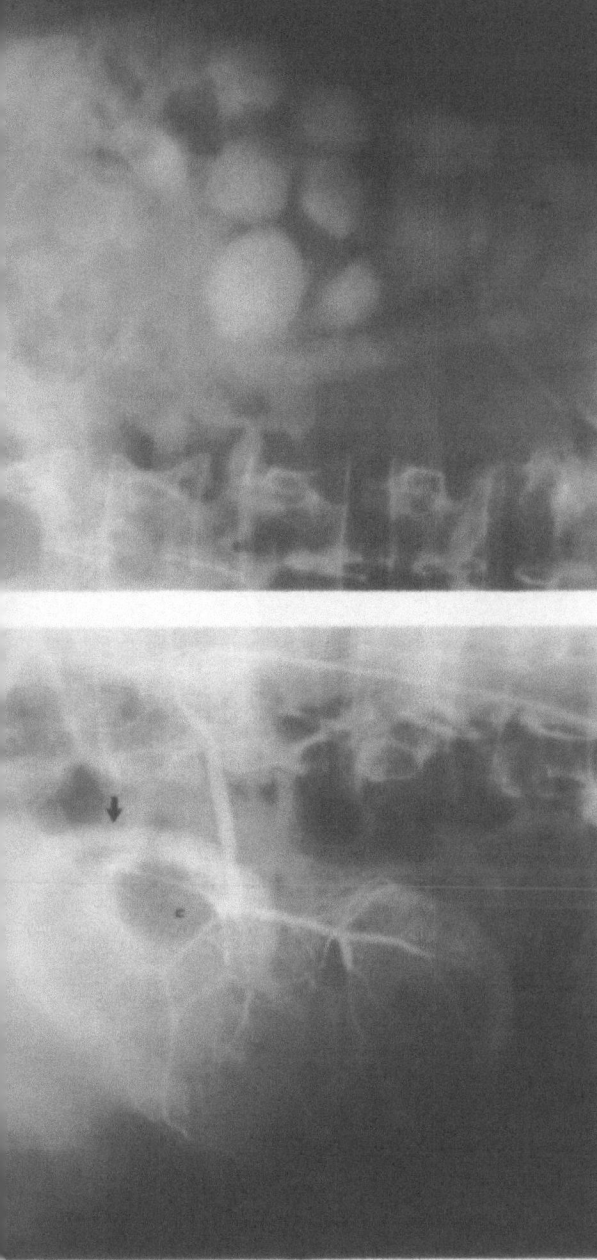

Figure 7.9. *Hydronephrosis. The IVU showed a non-functioning right kidney which was thought to be due to hydronephrosis resulting from a lower ureteric calculus. Selective arteriography shows marked displacement of vessels characteristic of hydronephrosis. Note the 'rim sign' (arrowed) due to the remaining functioning parenchyma. Note also the 'negative pyelogram' represented by large areas of translucent urine (n) instead of the normal dense pyelogram.*

Figure 7.10. *'Rim sign' in obstructive uropathy in an Egyptian male with shistosomiasis. The patient who has had a previous right nephrectomy was admitted with left loin pain and terminal haematuria. The high dose IVU shows a 15 cm kidney with multiple clubbed calyces against a translucent background (contrast-free urine in pelvis) and a compressed 'rim' of functioning parenchyma (arrowed). A subsequent retrograde proved the stricture.*

63

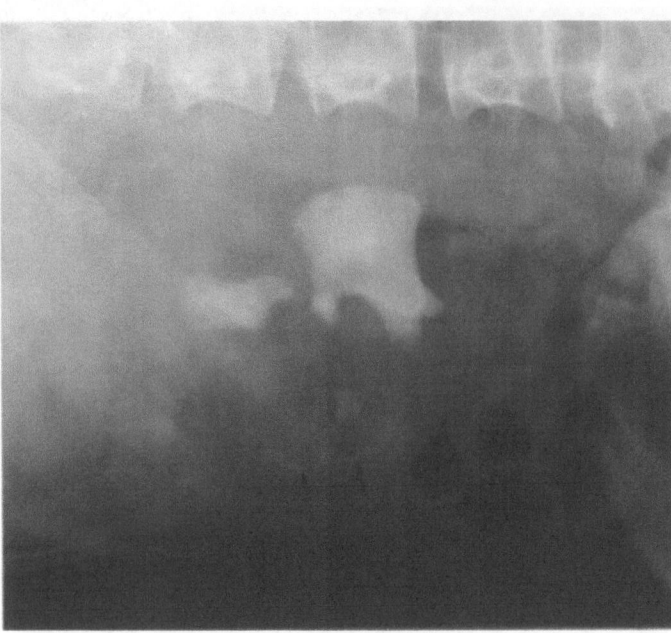

Figure 7.12. *'Crescent sign' in obstructive uropathy. Marked obstruction due to staghorn calculus, with remaining functioning parenchyma reduced to thin crescents (arrowed).*

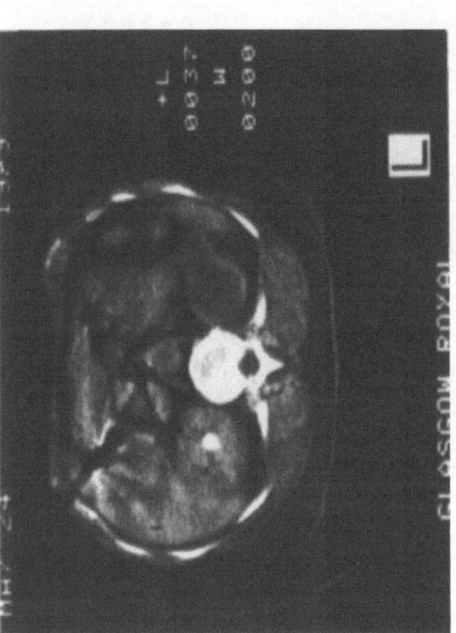

Figure 7.11. *CT scan of a hydronephrotic left kidney. Note the central hydronephrotic sac (h) with peripheral 'rim' of compressed parenchyma; k, right kidney; l, liver.*

the pelvicalyceal system, which may be represented by a 'negative' pyelogram (see Figure 7.9), and the remaining functioning parenchyma is represented by either a peripheral 'rim' of increased density (Figures 7.9, 7.10 and 7.11), or multiple 'crescents' (Figure 7.12), where the renal tissue is compressed around the dilated calyces. The ureter will show marked distension, and it will be dilated and tortuous.

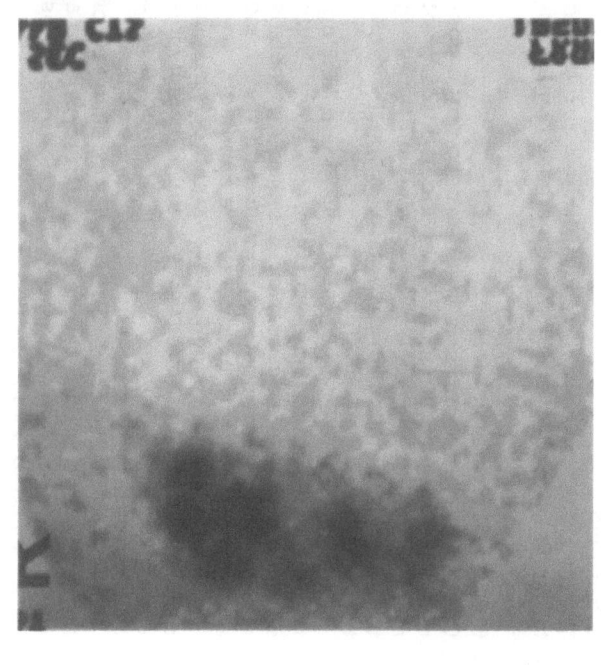

Figure 7.13 Obstructive uropathy due to ureteric strictures in shistosomiasis in a male from Upper Egypt. The right kidney has been obstructed for a long time and there had been diffuse atrophy with even reduction in the cortical thickness, as shown by the distance between the arrows (renal surface) and the dilated calyces. In this patient the left kidney had hypertrophied over this period but had recently become obstructed.

Figure 7.14. Renogram in a case of right-sided hydronephrosis in a patient with a previous left nephrectomy. This frame of a bolus renogram shows the isotope held up in dilated calyces, an appearance similar to calyceal filling on an IVU film (see Figure 7.13).

65

With very prolonged obstruction there will be a gradual onset of obstructive atrophy, with a progressive reduction in renal size and thinning of the renal cortex. The renal margin will be smooth (Figure 7.13).

Angiography in chronic obstruction will show a reduction in size of the renal artery, and there will be spreading of the intrarenal vessels (Figure 7.9).

Focal Postobstructive Atrophy

If there is localized obstruction due to a calculus in an individual calyx then there will, of course, be localized calyceal clubbing and shrinkage.

An unusual appearance which has been described in unilateral calculus obstruction is a diminished contrast density on the IVU, although the mechanism of this has not been fully explained.

Radioisotope Studies and Obstruction

The presence of a distended pelvis on an IVU examination or the absence of the third phase on a time/activity curve (renogram) are not definite evidence of an obstructive uropathy, although they strongly suggest it. To prove an obstructive uropathy there must be a positive result to a frusemide/water load IVU (Figure 1.5), or failure of descent after frusemide on a renogram.

The demonstration of an obstructive uropathy does not indicate an obstructive nephropathy. To prove this, abnormal parenchymal retention of a radiopharmaceutical must be shown, since the effect on the kid-

ney of an obstruction is to prolong the transit time through the parenchyma.

Isotope studies are useful in the postoperative follow-up of obstructive lesions (Figure 7.14).

Ultrasound

The distended calyces and pelvis will show as rounded transonic areas 'displacing' the compressed renal substance (see Figure 6.1).

Congenital Hydronephrosis

Congenital hydronephrosis is a not uncommon condition which usually presents in childhood but may not manifest itself until adult life. A characteristic feature in the history is that the pain is worse following the ingestion of large quantities of liquid.

Various anomalies such as mucosal folds, kinking, fibrous bands and aberrant vessels have been suggested as possible causes but it is likely that there is an underlying functional abnormality and that these anomalies, if present, exaggerate the condition.

Minor degrees of congenital hydronephrosis may be confused on standard urography with a flaccid hypertonic renal pelvis. Diuresis urography or renography is required to distinguish the two (see Chapter 1).

In the established condition there will be dilatation of the calyces and of an extrarenal pelvis. The pelvis has a convex lower margin and the pelviureteric junction has been likened to a wine glass.

8. Renovascular Disease

Renal hypertension can result from either parenchymal disease, for instance glomerulonephritis, pyelonephritis, interstitial nephritis, polycystic disease, collagen diseases, amyloidosis and bilateral obstructive uropathy, or renovascular abnormalities which are said to be responsible for approximately six per cent of hypertensive patients. The main causes of renovascular disease are atheroma and fibromuscular hyperplasia (Figure 8.1), but the other causes include trauma, aneurysms (Figures 8.1 and 8.2), neoplasms, external bands, angiomas, thrombosis and embolism.

Some years ago there was a vogue for operating on hypertensive patients with demonstrable renal artery lesions, but the results of surgery were disappointing and this, together with the increased effectiveness of antihypertensive drugs, has led to a considerable rethinking of the role of arterial surgery in hypertension. Routine intravenous urography as a screening procedure is no longer recommended, and should be reserved for those in whom there is other evidence of renal disease or for patients in whom it is thought

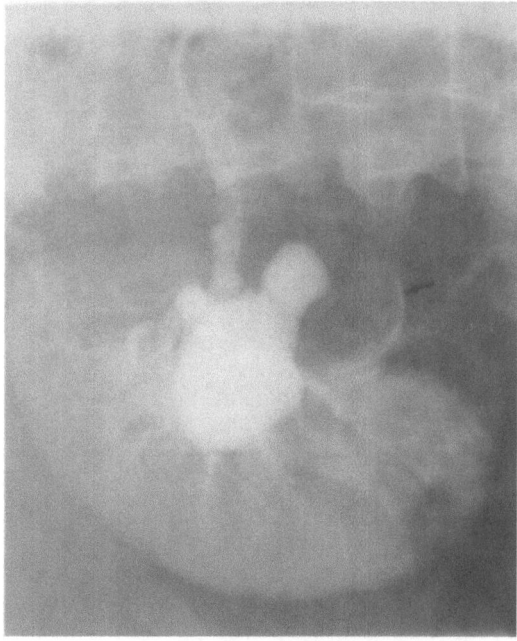

Figure 8.1. Aneurysm of renal artery and fibromuscular hyperplasia in a female under investigation for hypertension. The selective arteriogram shows a large renal artery aneurysm which is partly filled by a thrombus, as shown by the calcification (arrowed) outlining the full extent of the aneurysm. The fibromuscular hyperplasia characteristically affects the lateral extent of the vessel and shows irregular areas of narrowing and dilatation resembling a 'string of beads'.

67

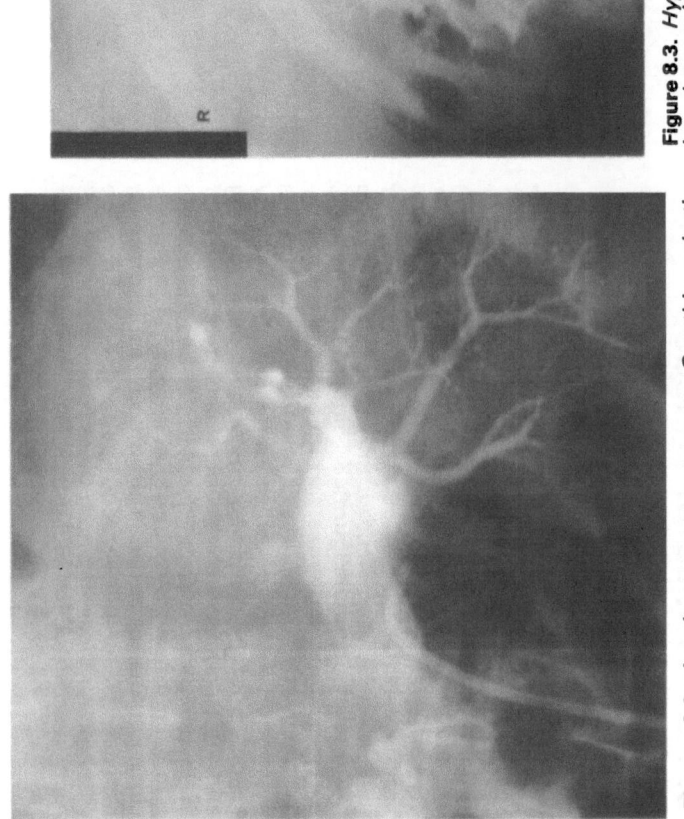

Figure 8.2. Arteriovenous aneurysms. On this selective arteriogram there are three upper pole aneurysms which are causing a massive arteriovenous shunt and early filling of the vein.

Figure 8.3. Hypertensive IVU in a female aged 42 years, who is a known hypertensive. The film shows a small dense pyelogram which followed a delayed nephrogram. There is also notching of the upper ureter caused by collapsed vessels. The arteriogram showed renal artery stenosis.

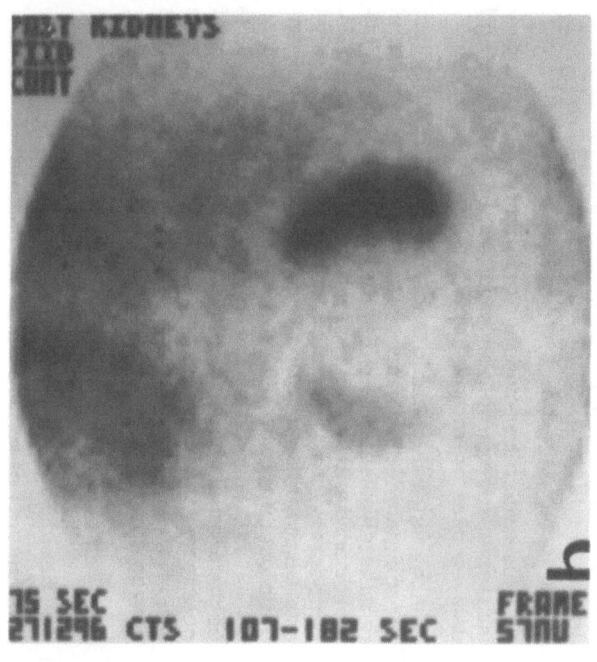

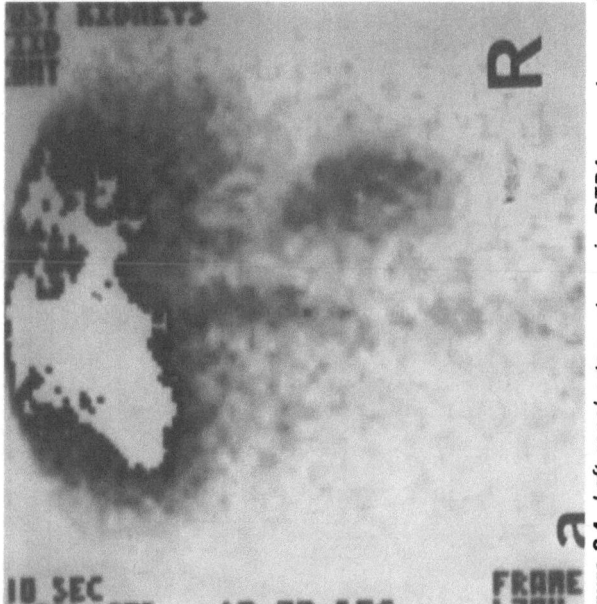

Figure 8.4. Left renal artery stenosis. DTPA scan in a patient whose IVU showed characteristic findings of renovascular ischaemia. (a) On the first frame (left) the radiopharmaceutical is present in the aorta and right kidney. (b) The later frame (right) shows the isotope to have reached the smaller less dense left kidney.

surgery would be appropriate. The latter would include:

1. Young hypertensives.

2. Patients showing a poor response to hypotensive agents or suffering from their side-effects.

3. Those with accelerated hypertension.

4. Those with other evidence of functional renal artery ischaemia, for example an impaired second phase and delayed peak on radioisotope activity/time curve.

The 'hypertensive (rapid sequence) IVU' will detect approximately 85 per cent of patients with unilateral renal artery disease, tending to miss those with bilateral disease and branch vessel disease (see Figure 8.3). Renography is an accurate method of assessing renal artery ischaemia and in many centres this is the screening procedure used (Figures 8.4 a and b, and 8.5).

If an IVU is used as the initial investigation and is positive, renal vein sampling, with branch sampling if necessary, should then be carried out to see if the lesion is functioning. At this stage arteriography can be carried out.

The Rapid Sequence IVU

The features of renovascular disease are:

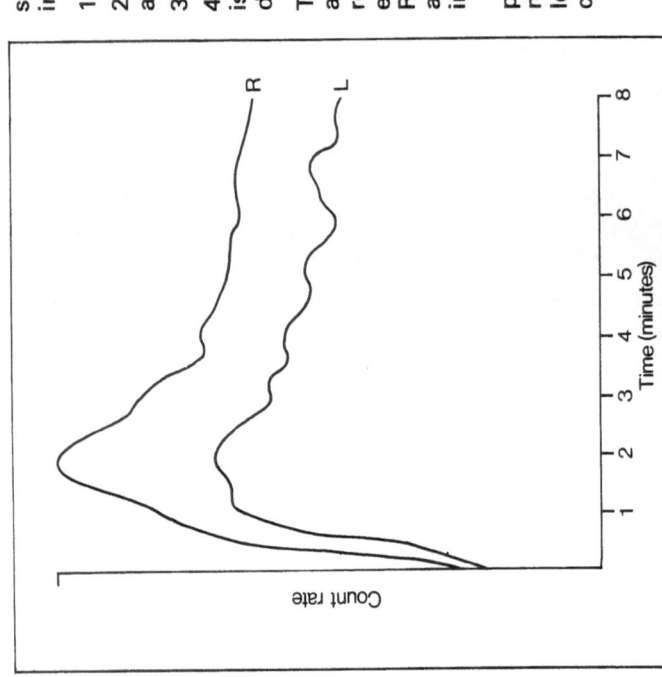

Figure 8.5. *The time activity curve in left renal artery stenosis, showing a reduced count rate on the left with a delayed flattened peak.*

1. A disparity in kidney length of more than 1.5 cm.
2. A delay in the pyelogram and nephrogram.
3. An increase in density of the pyelogram on the affected side.
4. Less distension of the pelvicalyceal system on the affected side.
5. Focal atrophy in segmental lesions.
6. Ureteral notching due to pressure from collateral vessels (see Figure 8.3).

It is most important to do an early sequence film, at one minute, to assess any delay in the appearance of the nephrogram. Although a delayed pyelogram will follow a delayed nephrogram if the earliest film is a 'five minute film' no conclusions about delay in excretion should be drawn.

Arteriography

A main stream arteriogram is carried out initially (Figure 8.6), both to assess lesions at the origin of the renal artery and also multiple renal vessels. If necessary, selective studies can be carried out for better definition of intrarenal vessels. Oblique views may be necessary to show narrowed segments.

The two principal causes of renal artery stenosis are:

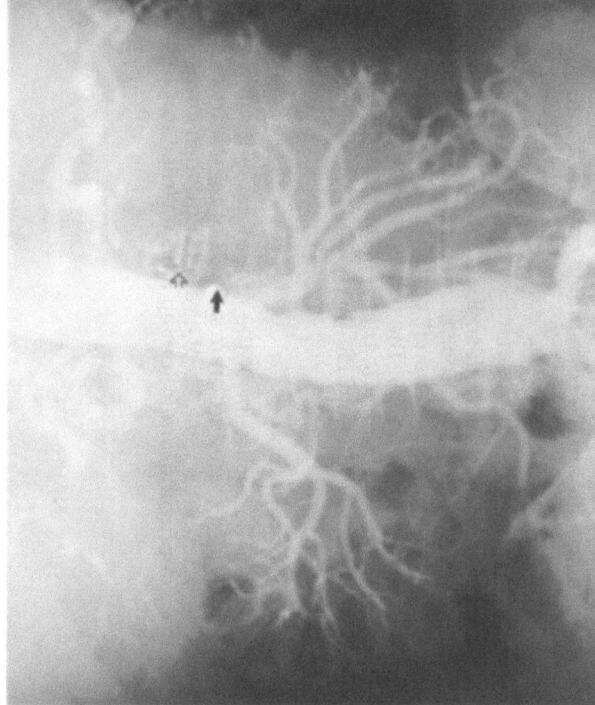

Figure 8.6. *Left renal artery stenosis. Mainstream aortogram shows generalized atheroma and block at origin of left renal artery (black arrow). A collateral circulation is seen (white arrow). The patient was a known hypertensive with delayed excretion on the left on the IVU.*

71

1. Atheroma, in which the lesion tends to be in the proximal third of the vessel and associated with diffuse atherosclerotic disease.

2. Fibromuscular hyperplasia (FMH) which occurs in three forms, intimal, medial and subadventitial and occurs more commonly in middle-aged female patients.

Renal artery stenosis is not uncommon in normotensive patients and, as pointed out above, it also occurs in hypertensive patients who do not have evidence of ischaemic renal disease. The IVU in these situations tends to be normal. A normal parenchymal retention function also excludes a renovascular cause, even with angiographic changes.

Aneurysms and Arterial Malformations of the Renal Artery

These lesions are uncommon and are usually congenital. Poststenotic aneurysms may occur in both fibromuscular hyperplasia and atheroma, and microaneurysms are seen in polyarteritis nodosa. If the aneurysms calcify, a characteristic curvilinear calcification is present. Giant, partially thrombosed, aneurysms may occur in FMH (Figure 8.1).

Traumatic arteriovenous malformations are not uncommon following renal biopsy (Figure 8.2). They are particularly amenable to catheter embolization.

The Cortical Rim Sign in Renal Infarction

Cases have recently been described where the 'rim sign' has resulted from extensive infarction of the kidney, but with a surviving renal cortex supplied presumably by capsular vessels. The rim sign on the nephrotomogram will be similar to that seen in obstruction, but ultrasound will distinguish the two lesions.

Computer Tomography

A quantitative assessment of the rate of development and density of the nephrogram can be obtained from the serial attenuation values of a rapid sequence computerized nephrotogram following a bolus injection of contrast.

9. Trauma

Plain Radiograph

Other evidence of trauma such as fractured ribs, a pneumoperitoneum, scoliosis, diaphragmatic elevation and bowel displacement may be present. The renal outline may be enlarged secondary to haemorrhage or oedema, or ill defined due to haemorrhage or extravasation.

Intravenous Urography

In cases of trauma an IVU should be carried out as soon as possible to assess renal damage and also the presence of and state of the opposite kidney.

If there is significant oedema, there will be a reduced renal flow and a decrease in the nephrogram and pyelographic density, with attenuation of the pelvicalyceal system. A haematoma will result in a 'mass effect', displacing the calyces if it is intrarenal or displacing the kidney if it is extrarenal (Figure 9.1). A localized nephrographic defect will result from an ischaemic area, and if there is extensive vascular or parenchymal

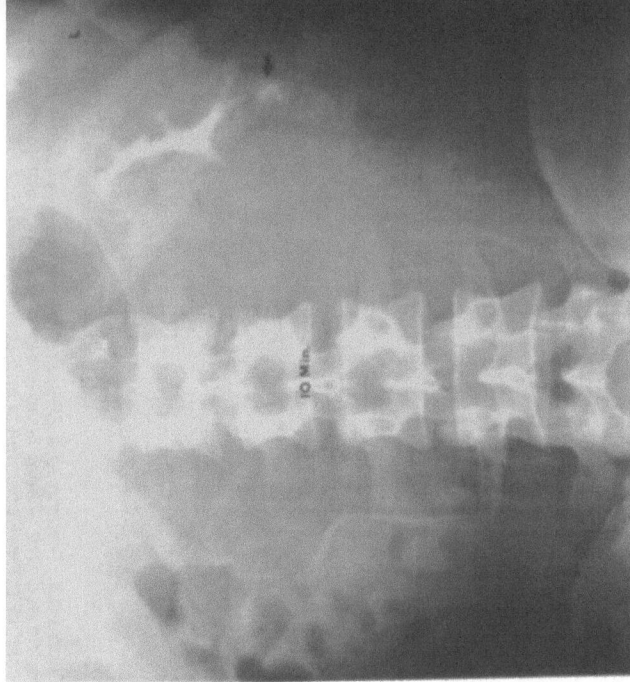

Figure 9.1. *The 10 minute IVU shows a leak of contrast from the lower pole calyx (arrowed). The lower pole of the kidney is displaced laterally by a haematoma.*

73

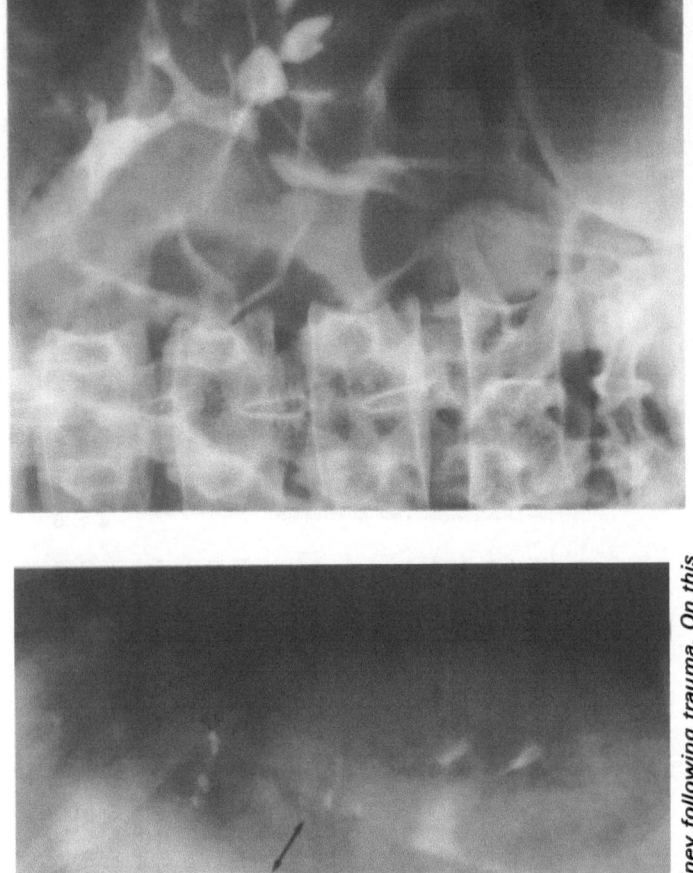

Figure 9.2. Rupture of left kidney following trauma. On this five minute IVU the left renal length is 19 cm (right = 14 cm) and there is an obvious laceration (double arrow). Contrast has leaked (open arrow).

Figure 9.3. Trauma in a 22-year-old male involved in a road traffic accident. There is an extensive blood clot forming a 'cast' of the calyces, pelvis and ureter.

injury there may be non-visualization.

Intrarenal, subcapsular or perinephric extravasation can result, depending upon the site of injury (Figure 9.1). Large lacerations in the kidney may be visible in the nephrogram phase (Figure 9.2). Blood in the pelvicalyceal system will present as a filling defect (Figure 9.3).

Angiography

The indications for angiography are:

1. Non-visualization on the IVU.
2. Non-diagnostic IVU.
3. Clinical deterioration.
4. Delayed haematuria.
5. A murmur.
6. Pre-operatively to assess the extent of injury, the vascular supply and the opposite kidney.
7. Late hypertension.

The contraindications are known allergy and a lack of time. Lacerations will be demonstrated (see Figure 9.4) and vascular lesions (such as arterial or venous thrombosis and arteriovenous fistulae) will be diagnosed. The intrarenal branches will be displaced by haematomata, which will result in a defect in the

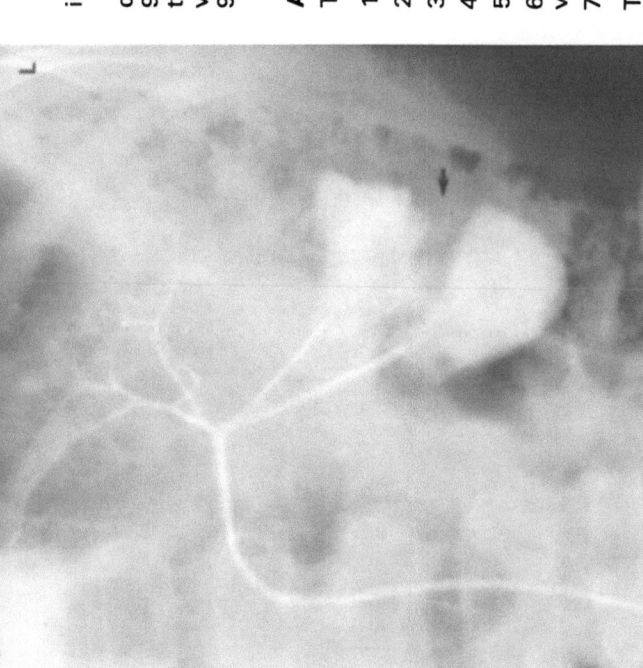

Figure 9.4. *Young boy involved in a road traffic accident. The selective left renal arteriogram shows stretching of the intrarenal branches due to a large haematoma. There is poor parenchymal perfusion of the upper pole. A large laceration is apparent in the lower pole (arrowed).*

75

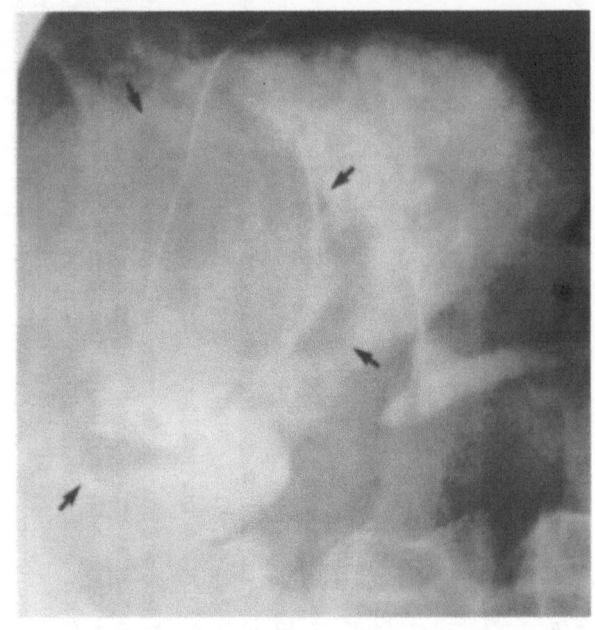

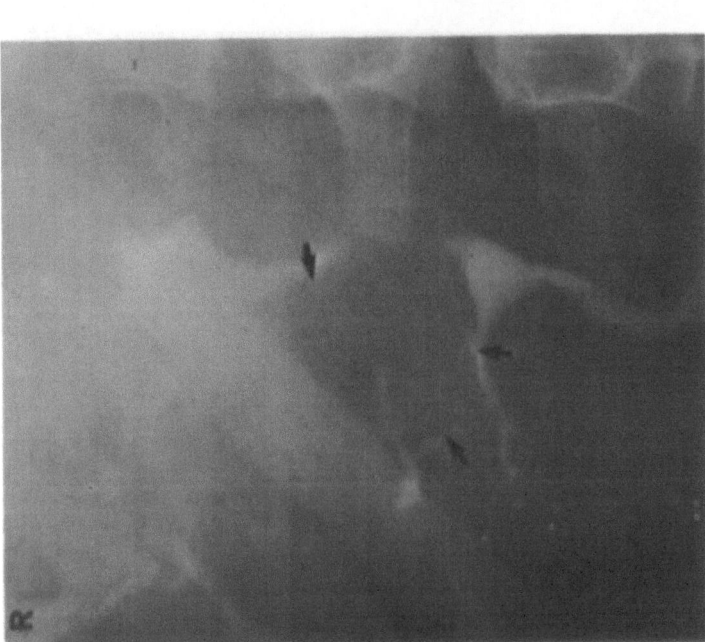

Figure 9.5 (a). Urinoma. IVU shows evidence of filling defect with displaced calyces. **(b)** Right selective renal arteriogram shows an avascular mass (arrows) in nephrogram phase. Ultrasound confirmed the cystic nature of the lesion, which at operation was found to be a urinoma.

nephrogram phase, and subcapsular haematomata will stretch the capsular vessels.

Radioisotope Studies

In the seriously ill patient, radioisotope studies are simple and quick to perform. They can provide evidence as to the vascular integrity and also give anatomical pictures which might reveal lacerations and non-functioning segments. Finally, an assessment of drainage can be made.

Urinoma

A urinoma or 'traumatic cyst' results when urine leaks out following trauma or calculus obstruction (Figure 9.5, a and b). The history is usually suggestive and the 'cyst' is investigated in the usual way.

10. Renal Transplantation and Osteodystrophy

Osteodystrophy

Renal osteodystrophy consists of osteomalacia (or rickets in children), secondary hyperparathyroidism and sclerosis. The contribution to the bony changes by osteomalacia and hyperparathyroidism varies from case to case, but osteomalacia tends to predominate in the milder cases and hyperparathyroidism in the more severe disease.

Rickets

The characteristic changes of rickets occur at the bone ends before epiphyseal fusion and consist of:

1. A widening of the zone of provisional calcification.

2. Fraying of the metaphyses which are widened to form a 'cup'.

If these changes occur in the ribs the so called 'rickety rosary' results. Secondary deformities, for example bowing of the limbs, may occur.

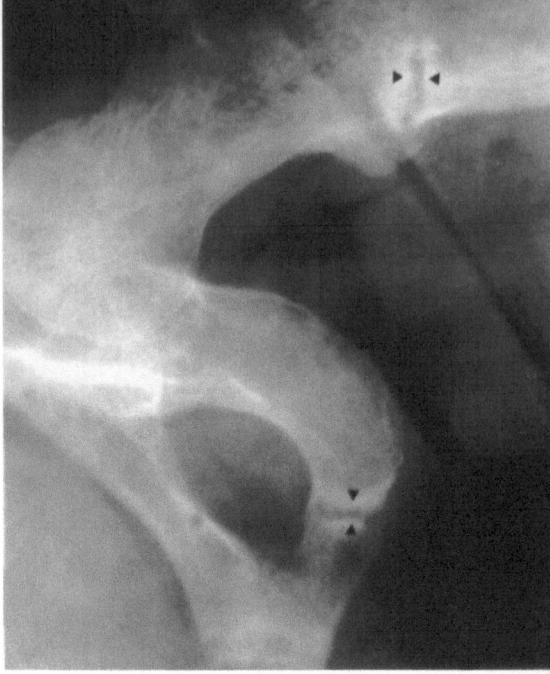

Figure 10.1. *Pseudofractures in osteomalacia. Adult female with renal osteodystrophy. There are two pseudofractures (arrowed), one of which crosses the inferior ischiopubic ramus and the other of which partly crosses the upper femoral shaft. Note the sclerotic margins bordering the translucent bands. There is a further fracture developing in the superior ramus, and erosion of the pubic symphysis.*

Osteomalacia

The reduction in bone density normally associated with osteomalacia tends to be masked by the presence of osteosclerosis and the predominant feature is the 'pseudo fracture' or Looser's zone. This consists of a thin lucent line, often with marginal sclerosis extending across part or the whole thickness of the affected bone (Figure 10.1). The lesions tend to be multiple and symmetrical, and occur at characteristic sites, that is, the long borders of the scapulae, the ribs, transverse processes, ischio-pubic rami, medial femoral necks and lesser trochanters, other long shafts and the metatarsals.

The earliest lesion may not be radiologically visible unless there has been slight collapse associated with the fracture, which will result in a thin dense line.

Secondary Hyperparathyroidism

Secondary hyperparathyroidism manifests itself in three main ways:

1. Subperiosteal cortical erosions: this appearance may be very widespread but frequent sites are the radial margins of the middle phalanges of the second and third digits (Figure 10.2), the ungual tips, the lateral ends of the clavicles, sacroiliac joints, symphysis pubis, ischial tuberosities, iliac crests, lamina dura and the temporomandibular joints.

79

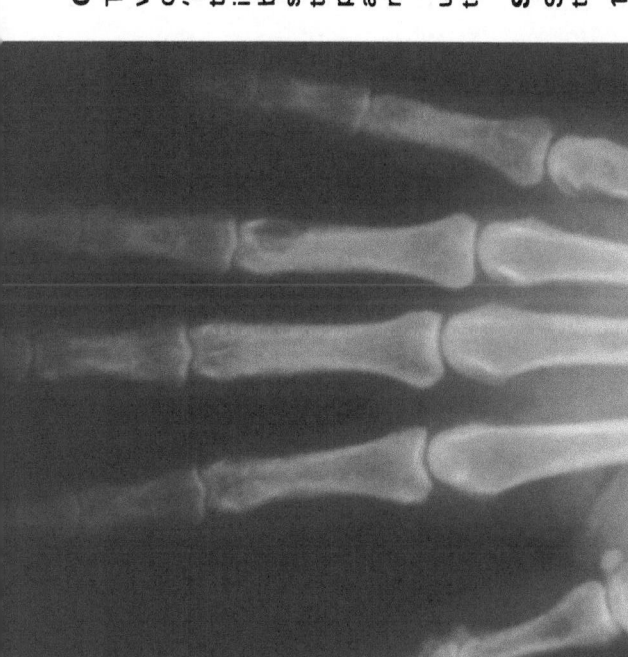

Figure 10.2. Hyperparathyroidism in renal osteodystrophy. Macroradiograph of the hand shows characteristic subperiosteal resorption affecting particularly the lateral borders of the middle phalanges and the ungual tips of the terminal phalanges. Note also the diffuse osteoporosis and 'brown tumour' in the metacarpal head.

2. Brown tumours: these commonly occur in the mandibles and facial bones, although again they may be present anywhere (see Figure 10.2). They are characteristically relieved by dialysis, provided that the serum calcium and phosphate are controlled. The large tumours characteristic of primary hyperparathyroidism do not normally occur.

3. Extraosseous calcification: this occurs typically in a periarticular distribution, in small vessels, particularly of the hands and feet (see Figure 10.3), and the subcutaneous tissues in the supraclavicular region. It is also seen in the breast, lung (see Figure 10.4) and the dura. Nephrocalcinosis, a feature of primary hyperparathyroidism, is not common in the secondary form.

Sclerosis

Sclerosis is best seen in the lumbar spine, where it is present as 'rugger jersey spine' (Figure 10.5).

Tertiary Hyperparathyroidism

Tertiary hyperparathyroidism is not unusual in long-term dialysis patients, and sampling of the neck veins with estimation of parathyroid hormone levels may be useful to localize the tumour.

Access Investigations

The normal route of access in dialysis patients is via an arteriovenous fistula or a vein loop. Shunts are often

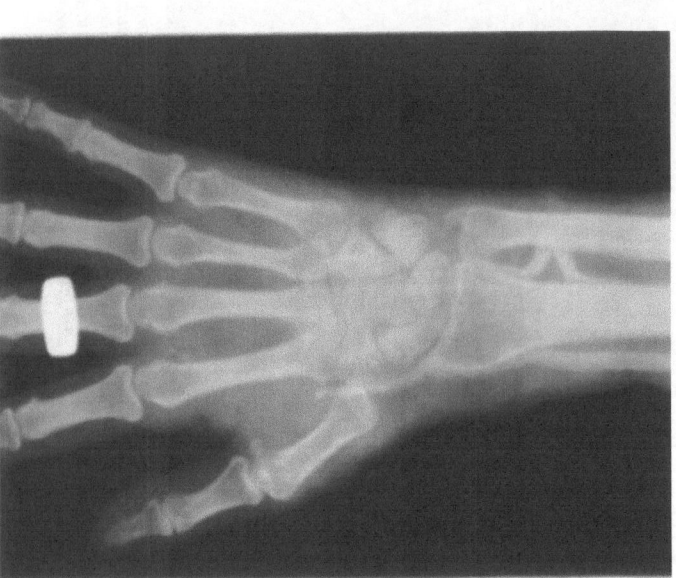

Figure 10.3. Vascular calcification in long-term dialysis. Note the marked Mönckeberg type of vascular calcification, particularly in the radial and ulnar arteries.

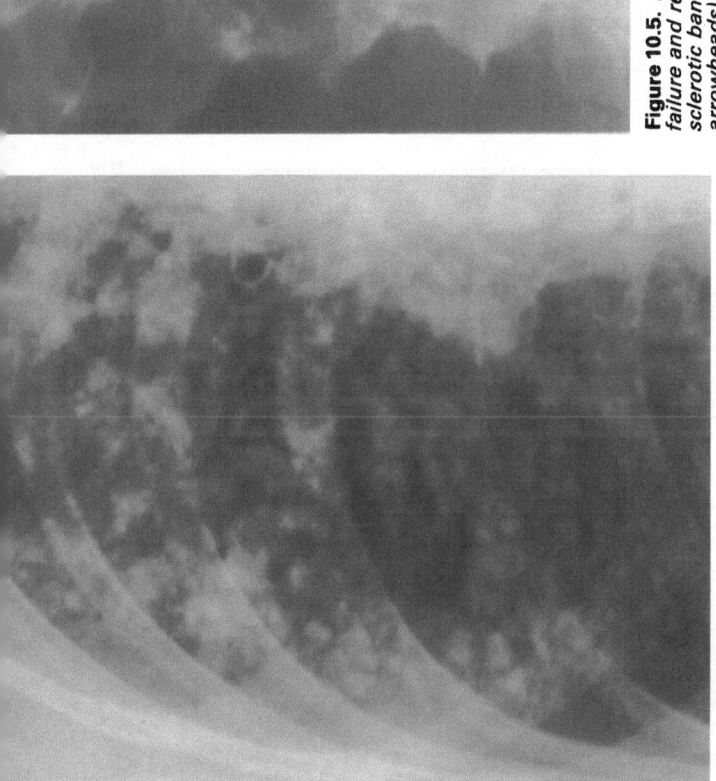

Figure 10.5. Rugger jersey spine. A female with chronic renal failure and renal osteodystrophy. The vertebral bodies have sclerotic bands across their upper and lower margins (open arrowheads) with intervening translucent bands resulting in a 'rugger jersey spine'. The curvilinear markings (black arrowheads) anterior to the spine are due to calcification in a bilateral tuberculous autonephrectomy.

Figure 10.4. Metastatic calcification in the lungs in a female patient with long-standing renal failure and hyperparathyroidism.

created as a temporary measure while the arterioven-ous links are being established.

Arteriovenous fistulae are frequently the site of thrombosis, localized vascular stenosis (see Figure 10.6), or longer areas of narrowing.

Traumatic arteritis is a common complication of shunts as well as narrowing at the shunt tip.

Renal Transplants

Complications

The main complications are:

1. Vascular: stenosis—particularly arterial.
2. Parenchymal: acute tubular necrosis; rejection.
3. Extrarenal: haematoma; lymphocoele; urinoma.

It should be remembered that there may be an increase in size of up to 20 per cent, due to compensatory hyper-trophy, if a small kidney is put in a large recipient.

Normal Isotope Studies

A normal isotope renogram (Figure 10.7) shows peak extraction of the radiopharmaceutical from the blood stream at eight minutes, with gradual clearing to the background level at 30 minutes.

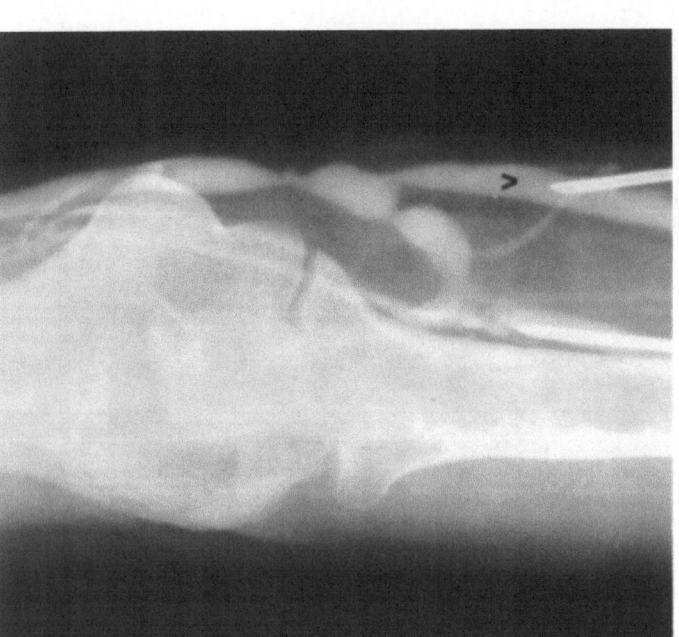

Figure 10.6. *Stenotic lesion at the termination of the venous end of an arteriovenous fistula, and in a vein draining the fistula; v, venous end.*

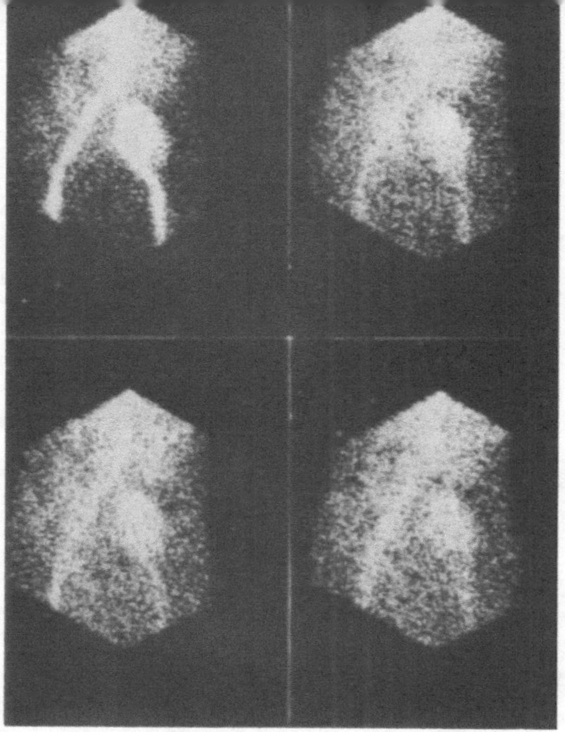

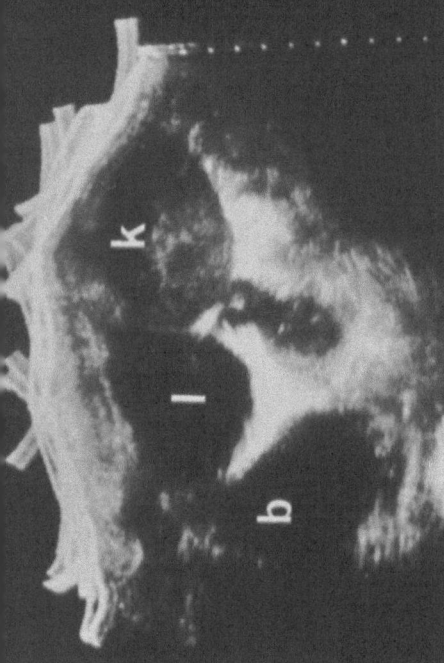

Figure 10.8. *Longitudinal ultrasound scan of pelvis showing a lymphocoele (l) associated with a renal transplant (k); b, bladder.*

Normal Angiogram

The catheter is usually introduced through the contralateral femoral artery to avoid damaging the anastomotic vessels, but if selective studies are required an ipsilateral approach may be used. Oblique studies may be required to show the anastomosis. Normally, there is clearance of the contrast from the kidney by the time the ileo-femoral vessels have cleared.

Figure 10.7. *Normal technetium radioisotope study of a transplanted kidney.*

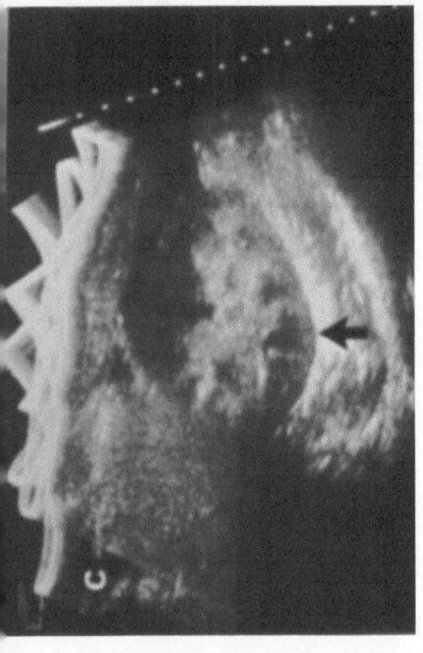

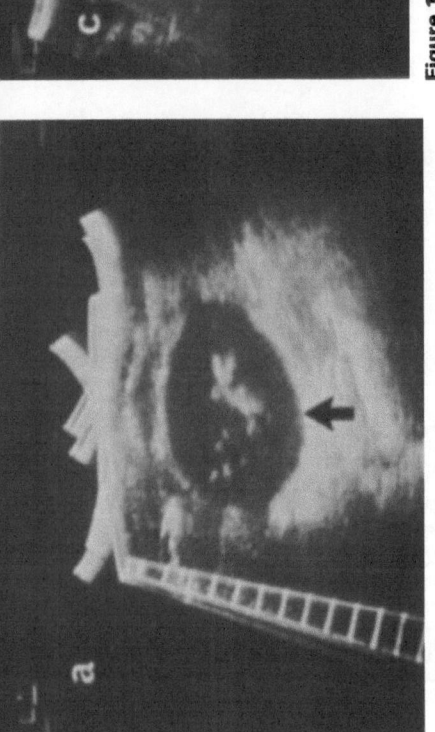

Figure 10.9 (a, b and c). *Serial ultrasound examinations in a rejecting transplant kidney (arrowed). These longitudinal scans show progressive enlargement and disorganization of the renal architecture.*

Rejection

Radioisotope Studies

Radioisotope studies are sensitive indicators of rejection and are normally carried out first. In early rejection there is delay in extraction and excretion of the radioisotope but a similar appearance will result from outflow obstruction and an IVU would then be

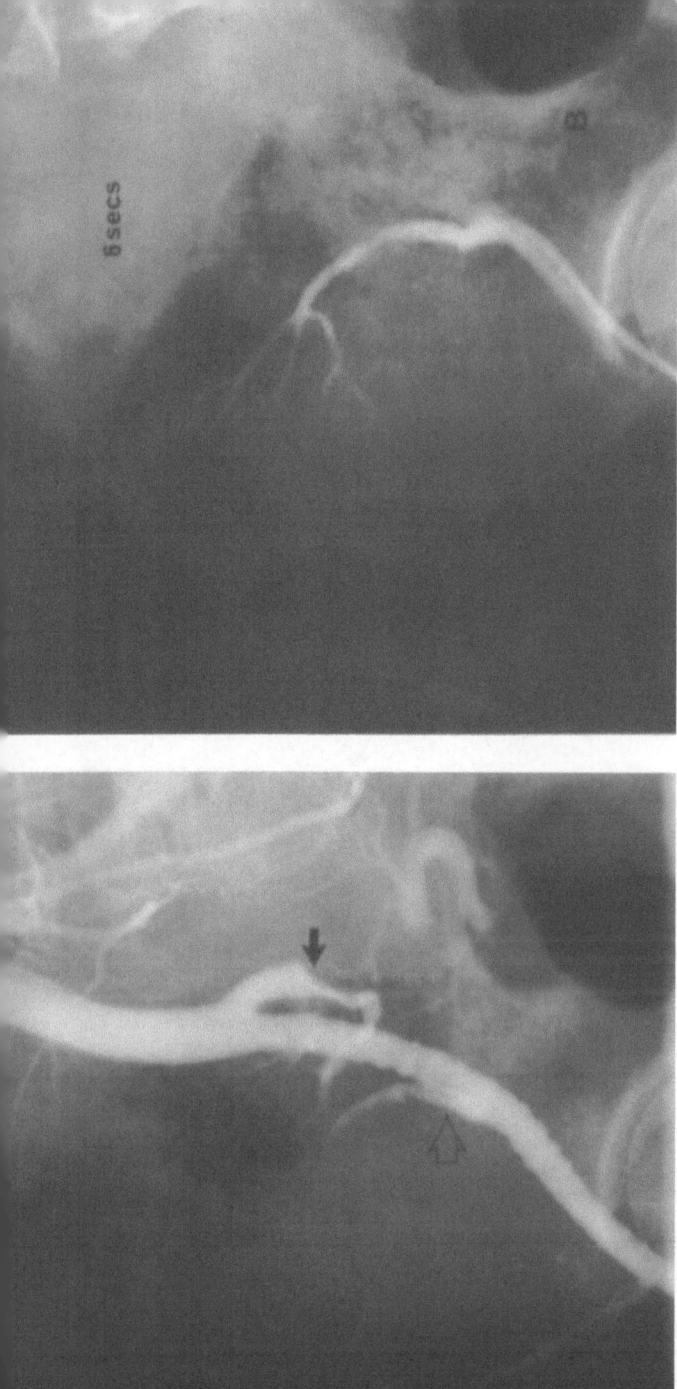

6 secs

B

Figure 10.10 (a and b). *Transplant rejection. A kidney with two renal arteries has been transplanted with an end-to-end anastomosis with the internal iliac artery (black arrow), and end-to-side anastomosis with the external iliac artery (white arrow). The mainstream injection (left) shows poor renal flow with only the main vessels outlined and narrowing at the upper anastomosis. The rippling is due to standing waves. Selective catheterization of the lower vessel (right) shows marked vascular pruning and delayed flow at 6 seconds.*

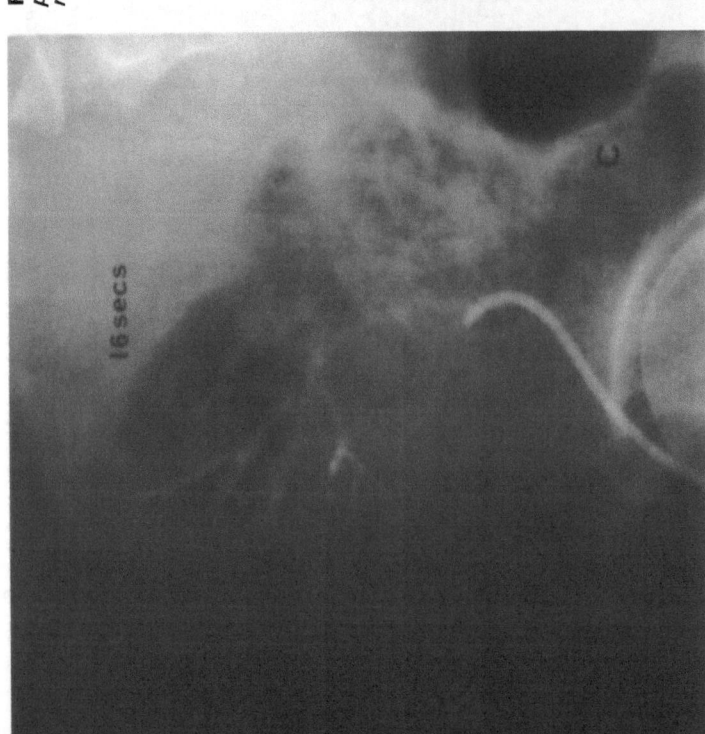

Figure 10.10 (c). Same case as Figure 10, a and b. Contrast persists in the vessels at 16 seconds indicating a markedly reduced flow.

necessary. With severe rejection the uptake of the radioisotope may be reduced to almost zero. In this situation the main differential diagnosis is renal artery stenosis, and angiography will be required. Renography can be carried out after the injection of frusemide when an obstructive lesion is suspected, in the same way as a frusemide/high dose IVU is performed.

An early reduction in renal perfusion, as well as function, suggests rejection. In acute tubular necrosis, perfusion will initially be maintained.

Ultrasound

Ultrasound is particularly useful for monitoring the progress of transplants as it is a non-invasive technique, and it can be used serially to assess the size of

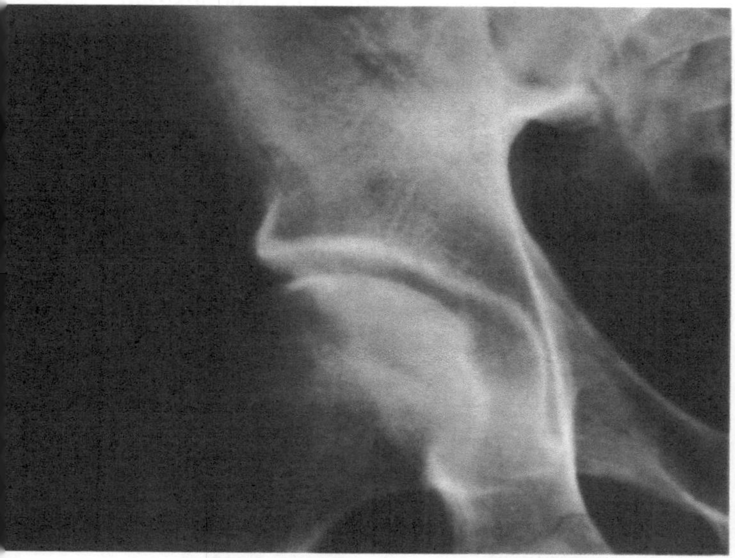

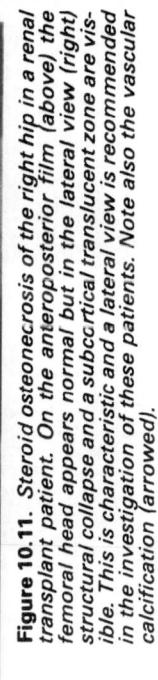

Figure 10.11. Steroid osteonecrosis of the right hip in a renal transplant patient. On the anteroposterior film (above) the femoral head appears normal but in the lateral view (right) structural collapse and a subcortical translucent zone are visible. This is characteristic and a lateral view is recommended in the investigation of these patients. Note also the vascular calcification (arrowed).

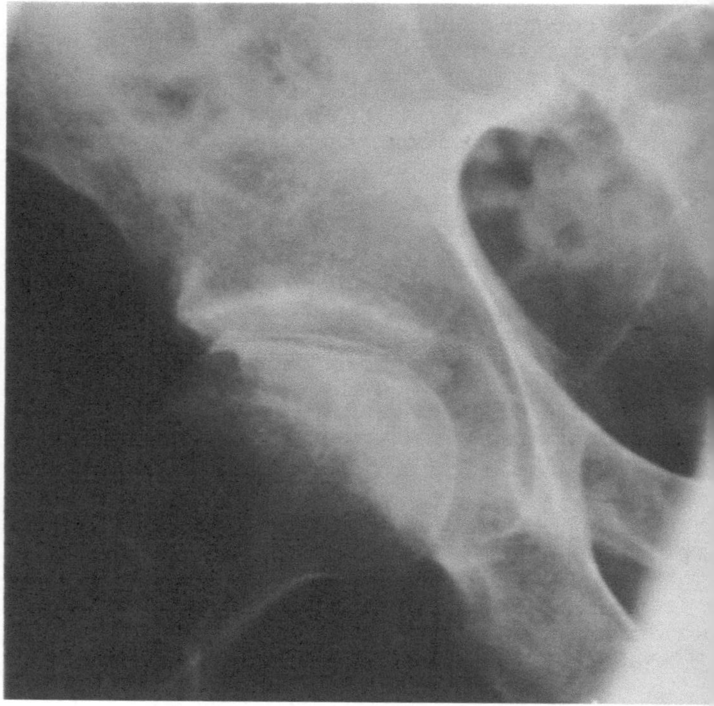

Intravenous Urography

The transplanted kidney can be assessed in the same way as a normal kidney by the standard IVU, but there is evidence to suggest that the injection of contrast agents in the early post-transplant period may precipitate a rejection. Many centres put clips on the kidney at operation to facilitate subsequent measurement of length.

Angiography

In the early phase of rejection there will be prolonged arterial transit time with stretching of the first and second degree arteries, reflecting the oedema, and non-visualization of the small arteries. The outline and nephrogram will be normal.

In severe rejection even the large arteries are not visualized well and no nephrogram phase will result. The renal outline will not be demonstrated (see Figure 10.10).

Steroid Osteonecrosis

Transplant patients on high dose steroid therapy are prone to osteonecrosis, which most commonly occurs in the femoral head (Figure 10.11).

Opportunistic Infection

Lifelong immunosuppression frequently gives rise to opportunistic infections, for example Pneumocystis carinii (Figure 10.12), and fungal infections.

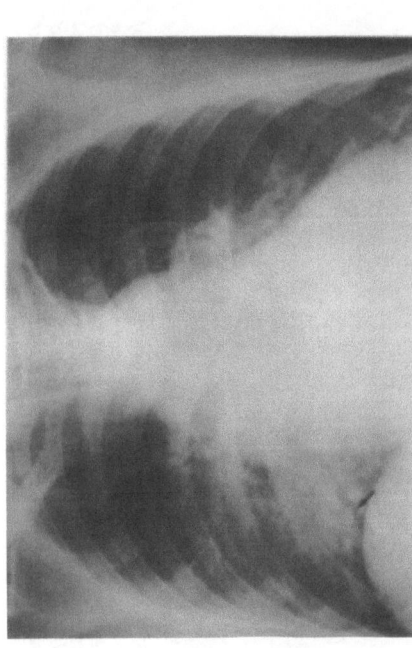

Figure 10.12. *Pneumocystis carinii in a transplant patient. There is bilateral consolidation sparing the upper zones, and an 'air bronchogram' is seen on the right (arrowed).*

the kidney, ureteric obstruction, and fluid accumulations associated with the transplant. The last group includes abscess, haematoma, lymphocoele (Figure 10.8) and urinoma. Ultrasound, as in the normal situation, can be used to guide an aspiration needle. A rejecting kidney will show a progressive increase in size and roundness which can be monitored by ultrasound (Figure 10.9, a, b and c).

Further Reading

Davidson, Alan J., *Radiologic Diagnosis of Renal Parenchymal Disease*, W. B. Saunders, London, 1977.

Emmett, J. and Whitton, *Clinical Urography (3rd edition)*, W. B. Saunders, London, 1971.

Hodson, C. J., Maling, T. M. J., McManamon, P. J. and Lewis, M. G., The pathogenesis of reflux nephropathy, *Br. J. Radiol.*, suppl. 13, 1975.

Kelsey Fry, I. and Cattel, W. R., The nephrographic pattern during excretion urography, *British Medical Bulletin*, 1972, **28**, 3, 227.

Saxton, H. M., Review article: Urography, *British Journal of Radiology*, 1969, **42**, 372–377.

Saxton, H. M. and Strickland, B. (Eds), *Practical Procedures in Diagnostic Radiology*, H. K. Lewis, London, 1972.

Sutton, and Grainge, *Textbook of Radiology*, 1975.

Index